Instructor's Guide & Testbank

MEDICAL TERMINOLOGY
WITH HUMAN ANATOMY
Third Edition

Jane Rice, RN, CMA-C
Medical Assistant Program Director
Health Occupational Instructor
Coosa Valley Technical Institute
Rome, Georgia

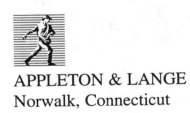

APPLETON & LANGE
Norwalk, Connecticut

Copyright © 1995 by Appleton & Lange
A Simon & Schuster Company

95 96 97 98 99 / 10 9 8 7 6 5 4 3 2 1

Prentice Hall International (UK) Limited, *London*
Prentice Hall of Australia Pty. Limited, *Sydney*
Prentice Hall Canada, Inc., *Toronto*
Prentice Hall Hispanoamericana, S.A., *Mexico*
Prentice Hall of India Private Limited, *New Delhi*
Prentice Hall of Japan, Inc., *Tokyo*
Simon and Schuster Asia Pte. Ltd., *Singapore*
Editora Prentice Hall do Brasil Ltda., *Rio de Janeiro*
Prentice Hall, *Englewood Cliffs, New Jersey*

ISBN: 0-8385-6272-8

PRINTED IN THE UNITED STATES OF AMERICA

ISBN 0-8385-6272-8

90000

9 780838 562727

TABLE OF CONTENTS

PREFACE

The paperwork necessary to run a class often consumes a great deal of an instructor's energy and time. This book is designed to sharply reduce that commitment, and help you, the instructor, keep your emphasis on teaching while using <u>Medical Terminology with Human Anatomy</u>, Third Edition. Here's what's included:

■ A complete SYLLABUS is provided for distribution to your class.

■ A PROGRESS SHEET allows students to maintain a record of chapters read, exercises and audio tapes completed, and post test results.

■ Specific test dates may be inserted into the TEST SCHEDULE, which may then be given to each student as a constant reminder of upcoming tests.

■ ANSWER SHEETS save you costly duplication of tests. One is provided for FORM A and another for Form B.

■ The TEST BANK is at the heart of the Instructor's Guide. Two post tests are provided for each chapter, Form A and Form B, and either may be copied straight from this book for easy administration. Each form is immediately followed by its answer key. Selection of form is at the discretion of the individual instructor. The advantages of supplying two forms are that the instructor may choose the test that best fits his or her own teaching style, and that an alternate test is readily available for student retakes. Two FINAL EXAMS and their answer keys are provided at the back of the Test Bank for the purpose of final testing.

SUPPLEMENTS

■ Upon adoption, a COMPUTERIZED TEST GENERATOR (IBM compatible) is available by contacting your local Appleton & Lange representative or by calling customer service at 1-800-423-1359. A menu-driven computer program designed to create examinations, it consists of <u>the same</u> test items included in this book, but provides the instructor with maximum flexibility due to the computerization of the material. The instructor can use the COMPUTERIZED TEST GENERATOR to quickly create tests either by choosing specific items or by having the program randomly select test items. Any test items in the pool may be previewed, and test items from one or more chapters may be included in the exam. Once selected, test items can be scrambled or left in order. If more than one chapter is chosen, test items may be shuffled or left grouped by chapter. Test items may be edited, deleted or added to the test item pool by the instructor with a special, easy-to-use text editor incorporated into the program. All technical questions regarding the program will be answered by Educational Software Concepts, Inc. at 1-800-748-7734.

- COMPUTERIZED STUDENT SELF-ASSESSMENT - Over 1,000 questions are provided in a multiple choice and fill-in-the-blank format. The learner is tested over material in a given chapter with the correct answer explained, as well as referenced by page number. A study plan is then generated from questions that were answered incorrectly. Study plans may be viewed directly on the computer screen or printed. COMPUTERIZED STUDENT SELF-ASSESSMENT GUIDES are available for purchase from Educational Software Concepts, Inc., 660 S. 4th Street, Edwardsville, Kansas, 66113, 1-800-748-7734. Instructors may receive a complimentary copy upon adoption.

- Upon adoption, the instructor can receive a COMPLIMENTARY THREE TAPE SET (45 minutes each side) of all the terms listed in the terminology sections. In order to facilitate learning, these audiotapes are available as an aid to pronunciation and understanding of the terms. Each term is pronounced, broken into its component parts, the definition of the part is given and then the term is pronounced again. By learning the component parts that are used to build medical words, one may easily acquire a working knowledge of medical terminology. These tapes are available for student purchase from Appleton & Lange at 1-800-423-1359 or by filling out the coupon found in Jane Rice's MEDICAL TERMINOLOGY WITH HUMAN ANATOMY, THIRD EDITION.

- Free to both the student and the instructor upon request is a single STUDENT TAPE which will contain two sides (thirty minutes each). The first side will focus on difficult terminology from three chapters: Integumentary System (Chapter 3), Endocrine System (Chapter 11) and Nervous System (Chapter 12). The "Tough Terms" will be pronounced and then defined. Side 2 will focus on key Spanish terms and short phrases. The term or phrase will be pronounced in Spanish, then defined in English. This offer is available through Appleton & Lange by filling out the coupon found in Jane Rice's MEDICAL TERMINOLOGY WITH HUMAN ANATOMY, THIRD EDITION. No telephone requests will be honored. Limit one per customer.

HOW YOU CAN BEST USE THIS TEXTBOOK

On the first day of class, introduce yourself, give an overview of the course, pass out the course syllabus, progress sheet, and test schedule. You may adapt these materials to suit the length of your course. For a 3 credit hour medical terminology course, cover the first two chapters of the text and then select eight other chapters that you wish to include. For a 5 credit hour medical terminology and/or anatomy course cover the first two chapters and then select the rest of the chapters according to any sequence that you choose.

It is important to cover Chapter 1 Fundamental Word Structure and then Chapter 2 The Organization of the Body using the information as it is presented in the text. Chapter 1 provides the basic building blocks necessary to the understanding of medical word structure. Chapter 2 provides basic information for understanding the organization of the human body.

KNOW THE BOOK THAT YOU ARE USING

I like my students to become familiar with their text so, on the first day of class, I ask them to turn to the back of the book. This is what they will find:

Appendix I Answer Key (pages 509-534) provides all the answers to the Learning Exercises and Review Questions for Chapters 1-18.

Appendix II Abbreviations (pages 535-544), includes over 850 abbreviations that may be used as a reference for common medical abbreviations, and medication and prescription abbreviations. On pages 542-544 are tables of weights and measures, and symbols that may be used as a reference for this course or a pharmacology course.

Appendix III Glossary of Component Parts (pages 545-551), contains all of the component parts that are included in the text (89 prefixes, 640 roots and combining forms, and 160 suffixes). These component parts will be learned according to the systems of the body or specialty area to which they relate. This is a definite bonus for individuals who take State Board Examinations, Certification Exams or Registry Exams, as they can use the component parts that they have learned and easily identify medical terms and their definitions in any given situation.

After the Glossary of Component Parts the student will find Flash Cards for the most commonly used prefixes, combining forms, and suffixes. These are provided in a cut-out format for the student to use as he/she studies medical terminology.

The last section of the text includes a General Index and a Spanish Index.

Now, have the students turn back to the beginning of the text and look at the Color Atlas. This atlas displays essential diagrams of the human body. This is a perfect complement to the discussion of the anatomy and physiology overview in chapters 2-16.

Example Teaching Plan: You may use this plan for chapters 3-16 of the text. I have selected The Endocrine System to give an example of how I use MEDICAL TERMINOLOGY WITH HUMAN ANATOMY.

CHAPTER 11 THE ENDOCRINE SYSTEM

ANATOMY and PHYSIOLOGY OVERVIEW

1. Reading Assignment-have the students read pages 281-290.

2. Discuss the anatomy and physiology overview. Have a "questions and answer" session. Show a videotape on the endocrine system. I use the Living Body Series from FILMS FOR THE HUMANITIES & SCIENCES, PO Box 2053, 743 Alexander Road, Princeton, NY 08540.

3. Ask the students to learn the chart that is on page 283. Discuss each endocrine gland and its primary functions.

4. Have the students learn the location of the various endocrine glands and be able to label the diagram that is on page 284. You can white-out the names of the glands, and then duplicate the drawing for student use.

5. Have the students complete the anatomy and physiology learning exercises, pages 304-305. After they have completed this section, have the students take turns and read a question and its answer.

6. You may select various endocrine glands and their hormones and have the student learn those that you wish to emphasize. If you are teaching more than a 3 hour course or using this text for anatomy and physiology you may choose to have the students learn more about each gland, the hormones produced, and their target areas.

INSIGHTS

For fun and additional information, have the students read the Insights-Diabetes Mellitus on page 291. Have a general discussion on this topic. You may wish to show a video on Diabetes. You can borrow a video from your local Diabetes Chapter or order one from numerous companies, such as MEDCOM/TRAINEX VIDEOTAPES 1-800-558-9595.

TERMINOLOGY with SURGICAL PROCEDURES & PATHOLOGY

1. Have the students learn the medical term, its component parts (part-definition), and then relate this knowledge to the definition of the term. Go over the first ten terms, and then play the Audiotape that goes with this chapter. Play the tape for approximately ten minutes and then stop the tape and review the terms that the students have heard. Each term is pronounced, then broken into its component parts and the part defined. Have the students do this. Resume playing the tape and repeat the same process of learning. A bookmark has been provided so that the student may use it to cover any one of the three columns in the terminology section. Also the flash cards can be used as the student learns the terminology. Students may wish to make additional flash cards as needed.

2. Have the students complete the Word Parts, Identifying Medical Terms, and Spelling Sections in the Learning Exercises, pages 305-308. After the students have completed this activity, go over it in class.

VOCABULARY WORDS

1. Go over the vocabulary words, pages 298-299 with the students. You pronounce the word, and then have the students say the word. You may have the students take turns, and read the definitions out loud . This is good practice. Naturally, you will help those who have difficulty pronouncing the terms in the definitions.

2. Have the students complete the matching section of the Review Questions, page 308. After they have completed this, go over it in class.

ABBREVIATIONS

Go over the abbreviations with the students. You may pronounce the definitions and/or have the students take turns and do this. I have selected ten abbreviations for each chapter test. I usually tell my students the ones that I would like for them to know. Have the students complete the abbreviations section on pages 308-309. After they have completed this section, go over it in class.

DRUG HIGHLIGHTS

You may wish to go over this information with your students and select portions that you want them to know, or simply use it as a reference.

COMMUNICATION ENRICHMENT

This new feature provides an opportunity for one to learn English and/or Spanish for selected general terms and medical terms associated with the subject of the chapter. This is an option for each student. Also, a free tape is available for the student. It provides an opportunity to listen to some of the Spanish terminology.

DIAGNOSTIC and LABORATORY TESTS

Go over this section with the students. Pronounce the test and have the students take turns and read the description. Have the students complete the Diagnostic and Laboratory Tests section, page 309 of the Review Questions. After they have completed this, go over this material in class.

LEARNING EXERCISES and REVIEW QUESTIONS

After the students have completed the Learning Exercises and Review Questions, I go around the classroom and check their work. On the Progress Sheet there is a work checked column, and I initial this, indicating that the student has completed his/her work. This is part of the daily grade and I average this in with the post test grades.

I make a copy of the learning exercises and review questions and cut these out and fold them and then put them in an envelope. As a review before testing, these questions are passed around and each student draws a question. The student reads the question out loud, and if possible answers the question. If the student does not know the answer, then another student may raise his/her hand and answer the question.

The first time you use this learning tool some students may be shy and not want to participate, but after the ice is broken, it can be a fun way to review.

I have found that if the students know the materials that are included in the Learning Exercises and Review Questions they generally do very well on the Post Test.

I hope that this example teaching plan will help you make the best use of MEDICAL TERMINOLOGY WITH HUMAN ANATOMY. Thank you for selecting this text.

Jane Rice

SYLLABUS

COURSE: Medical Terminology

INSTRUCTOR: _____

TEXTBOOK: MEDICAL TERMINOLOGY WITH HUMAN ANATOMY, Rice, Third Edition, Appleton and Lange, E. Norwalk, CT

OBJECTIVE: On completion of this course you will be able to analyze, build, spell, and pronounce medical words that relate to the human body, oncology, and radiology and nuclear medicine. You will identify and give the meaning of selected vocabulary words and abbreviations, and describe diagnostic and laboratory tests that are included in each chapter of the text. You will be able to describe each system of the body, stating its function(s), and its primary and accessory organs.

CONTENT:
- I. Fundamental Word Structure
- II. The Organization of the Body
- III. The Integumentary System
- IV. The Skeletal System
- V. The Muscular System
- VI. The Digestive System
- VII. The Cardiovascular System
- VIII. Blood and The Lymphatic System
- IX. The Respiratory System
- X. The Urinary System
- XI. The Endocrine System
- XII. The Nervous System
- XIII. The Ear
- XIV. The Eye
- XV. The Female Reproductive System
- XVI. The Male Reproductive System
- XVII. Oncology
- XVIII. Radiology and Nuclear Medicine

REQUIREMENTS:
1. Students are required to attend class.
2. Students are required to complete daily/weekly learning activities as scheduled.
3. Students are encouraged to take test as scheduled. In the event that you are absent on test day, a makeup test will be given on the day that you return to class. This test will be different from the one given on test day.

EVALUATION:
1. Daily grades and chapter post tests will count as 2/3 of the grade.
2. The final examination will count as 1/3 of the grade.

PROGRESS SHEET
Medical Terminology

	Chapter Read	Learning Exercises Completed	Listened to Audiotape	Work Checked	Post Test
Chapter 1.	_____	_____	_____	_____	_____
Chapter 2.	_____	_____	_____	_____	_____
Chapter 3.	_____	_____	_____	_____	_____
Chapter 4.	_____	_____	_____	_____	_____
Chapter 5.	_____	_____	_____	_____	_____
Chapter 6.	_____	_____	_____	_____	_____
Chapter 7.	_____	_____	_____	_____	_____
Chapter 8.	_____	_____	_____	_____	_____
Chapter 9.	_____	_____	_____	_____	_____
Chapter 10.	_____	_____	_____	_____	_____
Chapter 11.	_____	_____	_____	_____	_____
Chapter 12.	_____	_____	_____	_____	_____
Chapter 13.	_____	_____	_____	_____	_____
Chapter 14.	_____	_____	_____	_____	_____
Chapter 15.	_____	_____	_____	_____	_____
Chapter 16.	_____	_____	_____	_____	_____
Chapter 17.	_____	_____	_____	_____	_____
Chapter 18.	_____	_____	_____	_____	_____

NAME_____

DATE_____

GRADE_____

TEST DATE SCHEDULE
Medical Terminology

Scheduled Test Date	Chapter Heading
_____	Fundamental Word Structure
_____	The Organization of the Body
_____	The Integumentary System
_____	The Skeletal System
_____	The Muscular System
_____	The Digestive System
_____	The Cardiovascular System
_____	Blood and The Lymphatic System
_____	The Respiratory System
_____	The Urinary System
_____	The Endocrine System
_____	The Nervous System
_____	The Ear
_____	The Eye
_____	The Female Reproductive System
_____	The Male Reproductive System
_____	Oncology
_____	Radiology and Nuclear Medicine
_____	Final Exam

Daily Average _____   Name _____

Final Exam   _____   Date _____

Grade   _____

MEDICAL TERMINOLOGY
POST TEST A
ANSWER SHEET

NAME _____

DATE _____

TEST _____

1. _____
2. _____
3. _____
4. _____
5. _____
6. _____
7. _____
8. _____
9. _____
10. _____
11. _____
12. _____
13. _____
14. _____
15. _____
16. _____
17. _____
18. _____
19. _____
20. _____
21. _____
22. _____
23. _____
24. _____
25. _____

26. _____
27. _____
28. _____
29. _____
30. _____
31. _____
32. _____
33. _____
34. _____
35. _____
36. _____
37. _____
38. _____
39. _____
40. _____
41. _____
42. _____
43. _____
44. _____
45. _____
46. _____
47. _____
48. _____
49. _____
50. _____

MEDICAL TERMINOLOGY
POST TEST B
ANSWER SHEET

NAME _____

DATE _____

TEST _____

1. _____
2. _____
3. _____
4. _____
5. _____
6. _____
7. _____
8. _____
9. _____
10. _____
11. _____
12. _____
13. _____
14. _____
15. _____
16. _____
17. _____
18. _____
19. _____
20. _____
21. _____
22. _____
23. _____
24. _____
25. _____

26. _____
27. _____
28. _____
29. _____
30. _____
31. _____
32. _____
33. _____
34. _____
35. _____
36. _____
37. _____
38. _____
39. _____
40. _____
41. _____
42. _____
43. _____
44. _____
45. _____
46. _____
47. _____
48. _____
49. _____
50. _____

FUNDAMENTAL WORD STRUCTURE
CHAPTER 1
POST TEST A

PART I MULTIPLE CHOICE
DIRECTIONS: Select the best answer to each multiple choice question and write the appropriate letter on the answer sheet.

1. A syllable placed at the beginning of a word is called:
   a. suffix   c. prefix
   b. root   d. combining form

2. The foundation of a word is the:
   a. combining vowel   c. word root
   b. combining form   d. prefix

3. The prefix ab means:
   a. away from   c. near
   b. toward   d. far

4. The prefix dia means:
   a. double   c. across
   b. through   d. complete

5. The term antipyretic means:
   a. a state of fever   c. pertaining to against fever
   b. against heat   d. pertaining to against heat

6. The term _____ means a condition of feeling bad.
   a. lethargy   c. cahexia
   b. cachexia   d. cachet

7. A milliliter is:
   a. one-hundredth of a liter
   b. one-tenth of a liter
   c. one-millionth of a liter
   d. one-thousandth of a liter

8. A condition in which there is a death of tissue is:
   a. necrosis   c. necrose
   b. neurosis   d. nephrosis

9. A _____ is an instrument used to view small objects.
   a. macroscope   c. microscope
   b. microscopy   d. macroscopy

10. The process of being stuck together is:
    a. scar   c. abhesion
    b. adherent   d. adhesion

11. The prefix pro means:
    a. before   c. between
    b. after   d. within

12. The suffix _____ means the study of:
    a. logist   c. logo
    b. logy   d. logos

13. The suffix pathy means:
    a. disease   c. condition
    b. death   d. tissue

14. The suffix _____ means knowledge:
    a. gosis   c. gnoses
    b. gnosos   d. gnosis

15. The combining form onco means:
    a. cyst   c. growth
    b. tumor   d. swelling

16. _____ is the use of chemical agents to treat disease.
    a. Chemotherapy   c. Chemistry
    b. Chemotherapist   d. Chemtherapy

17. The prefix tri means:
    a. two   c. three
    b. six   d. seven

18. The suffix centesis means:
    a. surgical puncture
    b. surgical incision
    c. surgical excision
    d. surgical repair

19. To carry impulses toward a center is:
    a. abduction   c. afferent
    b. efferent   d. adduction

20. A chemical substance that destroys bacteria is a/an:
    a. virustatic   c. fungicide
    b. infectant   d. disinfectant

21. The term pallor means:
    a. grayish   c. blue
    b. paleness   d. yellow

22. _____ is the branch of medicine concerned with diseases of the skin.
    a. Dermatologist   c. Dermatology
    b. Dermalogy   d. Dermatosis

23. _____ is the branch of medicine concerned with diseases of the stomach and intestines.
    a. Entrogastrology
    b. Gastrenterlogy
    c. Gastroenterologist
    d. Gastroenterology

24. _____ is the branch of medicine that studies diseases of the eye.
    a. Ophthalmology
    b. Opthalmology
    c. Ophthalmologist
    d. Opthalmologist

25. The branch of medicine concerned with the aging process is:
    a. geriatrics
    b. geriatrician
    c. geratic
    d. geratrics

PART II MATCHING
DIRECTIONS: Using the answer sheet, write the letter of the definition that best matches the word.

26. antitussive
27. axillary
28. centigrade
29. diagnosis
30. diaphoresis
31. heterogeneous
32. etiology
33. neopathy
34. prognosis
35. thermometer
36. topography
37. triage
38. acute
39. malaise
40. malignant

A. A bad wandering
B. The sorting and classifying of injuries
C. Sudden, sharp, severe
D. A bad feeling
E. An agent that works against coughing
F. Pertaining to the armpit
G. Having 100 steps or degrees
H. A recording of a special place of the body
I. Determination of the cause and nature of a disease
J. The study of the cause(s) of disease
K. A unit of weight
L. Profuse sweating
M. Pertaining to a different formation
N. A condition of fore-knowledge
O. A new disease
P. An instrument used to measure degree of heat

PART III FILL-IN-THE-BLANK
DIRECTIONS: Using the answer sheet, write the correct abbreviation for each of the following.

41. _____ abnormal
42. _____ acute
43. _____ Celsius
44. _____ axillary
45. _____ biopsy
46. _____ computerized tomography
47. _____ discontinue
48. _____ diagnosis
49. _____ diagnosis-related groups
50. _____ family practice

FUNDAMENTAL WORD STRUCTURE
CHAPTER 1
POST TEST A

ANSWER KEY:

1.	c	26.	E
2.	c	27.	F
3.	a	28.	G
4.	b	29.	I
5.	c	30.	L
6.	b	31.	M
7.	d	32.	J
8.	a	33.	O
9.	c	34.	N
10.	d	35.	P
11.	a	36.	H
12.	b	37.	B
13.	a	38.	C
14.	d	39.	D
15.	b	40.	A
16.	a	41.	AB
17.	c	42.	AC
18.	a	43.	C
19.	c	44.	Ax
20.	d	45.	Bx
21.	b	46.	CT
22.	c	47.	D/C
23.	d	48.	diag, Dx
24.	a	49.	DRGs
25.	a	50.	FP

FUNDAMENTAL WORD STRUCTURE
CHAPTER 1
POST TEST B

PART I WORD PARTS
DIRECTIONS: Using the answer sheet, write the letter of the definition that best matches the word part.

1. a		A.	bad
2. ab		B.	small
3. anti		C.	process
4. auto		D.	surgical puncture
5. dia		E.	many, much
6. mal		F.	without
7. micro		G.	recording
8. milli		H.	beside
9. multi		I.	together
10. neo		J.	away from
11. para		K.	through
12. pro		L.	pertaining to
13. syn		M.	self
14. tri		N.	before
15. adhes		O.	knowledge
16. axill		P.	against
17. chemo		Q.	new
18. macro		R.	one-thousandth
19. necr		S.	stuck to
20. pyro		T.	center
21. -al		U.	heat, fire
22. -centesis		V.	three
23. -gnosis		W.	death
24. -graphy		X.	chemical
25. -ion		Y.	armpit
		Z.	large

PART II FILL-IN-THE-BLANK
DIRECTIONS: Using the answer sheet, write the correct abbreviation or meaning for each of the following.

26. abnormal		31.	gram
27. ac		32.	Gyn
28. Bx		33.	liter
29. Dx		34.	mL
30. D/C		35.	DRGs

PART III MULTIPLE CHOICE
DIRECTIONS: Select the best answer to each multiple choice question and write the appropriate letter on the answer sheet.

36. A _____ is a word or word element from which other words are formed.
    a. prefix   c. root
    b. combining form   d. suffix

37. The study of the cause(s) of disease is called:
    a. diagnosis   c. prognosis
    b. etiology   d. prognostication

38. A relationship of understanding between two individuals, especially between the patient and the physician is called:
    a. empathy   c. apathy
    b. afferent   d. rapport

39. _____ is the branch of medicine concerned with diseases caused by the action of antibodies to antigens.
    a. Epidemiology   c. Allergy/Immunology
    b. Endocrinology   d. Infectious disease

40. _____ is the branch of medicine concerned with the aspects of aging.
    a. Geriatrician   c. Geratic
    b. Geriatrics   d. Geratrics

41. _____ is the branch of medicine that studies the diseases of the eye.
    a. Ophthalmology   c. Opthalmology
    b. Otology   d. Otorhinolaryngology

42. A/an _____ is an agent that works against coughing.
    a. antiseptic   c. antitussive
    b. antipyretic   d. antidote

43. To carry impulses toward the center is:
    a. abduction   c. afferent
    b. efferent   d. adduction

44. The term pallor means:
    a. grayish   c. blue
    b. paleness   d. yellow

45. _____ means sudden, sharp, severe.
    a. Acute   c. Chronic
    b. Triage   d. Abate

46. A combination of signs and symptoms occurring together that characterize a specific disease is called:
   a. prognosis   c. diagnosis
   b. etiology   d. syndrome

47. The medical term for profuse sweating is:
   a. diphoresis   c. diaphoresis
   b. dyphoresis   d. diahoresis

48. A condition of death of tissue is called:
   a. neopathy   c. neurosis
   b. necrosis   d. neopaty

49. The rapid, widespread occurrence of an infectious disease is:
   a. epidemic   c. endemic
   b. prodemic   d. andemic

50. The process of cutting into is:
   a. excision   c. incision
   b. -ectomy   d. incise

FUNDAMENTAL WORD STRUCTURE
CHAPTER 1
POST TEST B

ANSWER KEY:

1.	F	26.	AB
2.	J	27.	acute
3.	P	28.	biopsy
4.	M	29.	diagnosis
5.	K	30.	discontinue
6.	A	31.	g, Gm
7.	B	32.	gynecology
8.	R	33.	L
9.	E	34.	milliliter
10.	Q	35.	diagnosis related groups
11.	H	36.	c
12.	N	37.	b
13.	I	38.	d
14.	V	39.	c
15.	S	40.	b
16.	Y	41.	a
17.	X	42.	c
18.	Z	43.	c
19.	W	44.	b
20.	U	45.	a
21.	L	46.	d
22.	D	47.	c
23.	O	48.	b
24.	G	49.	a
25.	C	50.	c

THE ORGANIZATION OF THE BODY
CHAPTER 2
POST TEST A

PART I MULTIPLE CHOICE
DIRECTIONS: Select the best answer to each multiple choice
question and write the appropriate letter on the answer sheet.

1. _____ tissue is the most wide-spread and abundant
   of the four body tissues.
   a. Epithelial   c. Muscle
   b. Connective   d. Nerve

2. The term proximal means:
   a. nearest the point of attachment
   b. away from the point of attachment
   c. opposite the point of attachment
   d. distal to the point of attachment

3. The _____ plane divides the body into superior and
   inferior portions:
   a. coronal   c. frontal
   b. midsagittal   d. transverse

4. The prefix ambi means:
   a. double   c. both
   b. two   d. one

5. The prefix homeo means:
   a. similar   c. unequal
   b. different   d. equal

6. The term somatotrophic means:
   a. to decrease the process of body growth
   b. stimulation of body growth
   c. formation of the body
   d. destruction of the body

7. _____ means the removal of water away from the body.
   a. Diffusion   c. Dehydrate
   b. Osmosis   d. Diaphoresis

8. The study of tissue is known as:
   a. pathology   c. pathologist
   b. histologist   d. histology

9. Fatty tissue throughout the body is called:
   a. celluloid   c. liposis
   b. adipose   d. sebosis

10. _____ is a slender physical body form.
    a. Endomorph   c. Ectomorph
    b. Mesomorph   d. Pseudomorph

11. The term cephalad means:
    a. away from the head   c. headache
    b. toward the head   d. pertaining to the head

12. The term inguinal means:
    a. pertaining to the flank
    b. pertaining to the abdomen
    c. pertaining to the back
    d. pertaining to the groin

13. The hereditary unit which transmits and determines one's characteristics or hereditary traits is the:
    a. gamete   c. gene
    b. gonad   d. genion

14. The _____ system consists of the skin and its appendages.
    a. intergumentary   c. cutaneous
    b. integumentary   d. subcutaneous

15. The _____ cavity is the space in the skull containing the brain.
    a. cranial   c. spinal
    b. thoracic   d. abdominal

16. The suffix tomy means:
    a. excision   c. section
    b. incision   d. puncture

17. In the term topical, -al means:
    a. pertaining to   c. related to
    b. pretaining to   d. action

18. In the term android, -oid means:
    a. form   c. like
    b. resemble   d. body

19. In the term mesomorph, -morph means:
    a. form   c. like
    b. resemble   d. body

20. _____ means pertaining to one side.
    a. Bilateral   c. Medial
    b. Lateral   d. Unilateral

21. _____ means pertaining to body organs enclosed within a cavity, especially the abdominal organs.
    a. Visceral   c. Peritoneal
    b. Inguinal   d. Ventral

22. In the anatomical position, the palms are:
    a. to the back   c. to the side
    b. to the front   d. to the middle

23. The _____ plane divides the body into anterior and posterior portions.
    a. midsagittal   c. coronal
    b. transverse   d. horizontal

24. The _____ plane vertically divides the body into right and left halves.
    a. midsagittal   c. coronal
    b. transverse   d. horizontal

25. _____ means towards the back.
    a. Anterior   c. Ventral
    b. Distal   d. Posterior

PART II MATCHING
DIRECTIONS: Using the answer sheet, write the letter of the definition that best matches the word.

26. caudal
27. apex
28. cilia
29. lateral
30. proximal
31. superficial
32. systemic
33. vertex
34. skull
35. nose
36. breast
37. armpit
38. finger
39. navel
40. hip

A. umbilicus
B. mammary
C. the top or highest point
D. pertaining to the tail
E. coxa
F. the pointed end of a cone-shaped structure
G. axillary
H. nearest the center
I. pertaining to the side
J. hairlike processes
K. pertaining to the surface
L. phalanx
M. pertaining to the body as a whole
N. rhino
O. cranial
P. cephalo

17

PART III FILL-IN-THE-BLANK
DIRECTIONS: Using the answer sheet, write the correct abbreviation for each of the following.

41. _____ abdomen
42. _____ anatomy and physiology
43. _____ anterior-posterior
44. _____ central nervous system
45. _____ cardiovascular
46. _____ gastrointestinal
47. _____ lateral
48. _____ respiratory
49. _____ endoplasmic reticulum
50. _____ posterior-anterior

THE ORGANIZATION OF THE BODY
CHAPTER 2
POST TEST A

ANSWER KEY:

1.	b	26.	D
2.	a	27.	F
3.	d	28.	J
4.	c	29.	I
5.	a	30.	H
6.	b	31.	K
7.	c	32.	M
8.	d	33.	C
9.	b	34.	O
10.	c	35.	N
11.	b	36.	B
12.	d	37.	G
13.	c	38.	L
14.	b	39.	A
15.	a	40.	E
16.	b	41.	abd
17.	a	42.	A&P
18.	b	43.	AP
19.	a	44.	CNS
20.	d	45.	CV
21.	a	46.	GI
22.	b	47.	lat
23.	c	48.	resp
24.	a	49.	ER
25.	d	50.	PA

PART I WORD PARTS
DIRECTIONS: Using the answer sheet, write the letter of the definition that best matches the word part.

1. ambi		A.	outside
2. ana		B.	first
3. bi		C.	study of
4. chromo		D.	body
5. de		E.	both
6. ecto		F.	fat
7. endo		G.	man
8. homeo		H.	color
9. meso		I.	resemble
10. proto		J.	control
11. uni		K.	tissue
12. adip		L.	up
13. andr		M.	water
14. cyt		N.	within
15. histo		O.	disease
16. hydr		P.	two
17. karyo		Q.	nature
18. patho		R.	middle
19. physio		S.	use, action
20. -ate		T.	excision
21. -logy		U.	down
22. -oid		V.	one
23. -some		W.	incision
24. -stasis		X.	similar
25. -tomy		Y.	cell
		Z.	cell's nucleus

PART II FILL-IN-THE-BLANK
DIRECTIONS: Using the answer sheet, write the correct abbreviation or meaning for each of the following.

26. abdomen	31.	CNS
27. A & P	32.	respiratory
28. AP	33.	gastrointestinal
29. lateral	34.	ER
30. cardiovascular	35.	PA

PART III MULTIPLE CHOICE
DIRECTIONS: Select the best answer to each multiple choice
question and write the appropriate letter on the answer sheet.

36. Hairlike processes that project from epithelial cells are:
    a. centrioles   c. cillia
    b. villi   d. cilia

37. _____ is the top or highest point.
    a. Vertex   c. Caudal
    b. Cortex   d. Cephalad

38. _____ is the physical appearance or type of makeup of an individual.
    a. Human genome   c. Phenotype
    b. Ectomorph   d. Endomorph

39. The component part for head is called:
    a. cephalo   c. carpo
    b. cranio   d. cervico

40. The component part for eye is called:
    a. ocluo   c. oto
    b. oculo   d. naso

41. The component part for arm is called:
    a. oro   c. brachi
    b. oto   d. buco

42. The substance within the cell's nucleus is called:
    a. karyoplasm   c. cytoplasm
    b. protoplasm   d. endoplasm

43. A/An _____ is a grouping of similar cells that together perform specialized functions.
    a. system   c. tissue
    b. organ   d. organelle

44. The measurement of the human body is called:
    a. anthropometry   c. physiology
    b. anatomy   d. antropometry

45. The most widespread and abundant of the body's tissue is:
    a. epithelial   c. muscle
    b. connective   d. nerve

46. _____ is nearest the point of attachment.
    a. Distal   c. Proximal
    b. Ventral   d. Dorsal

47. _____ is toward the back.
    a. Superior   c. Cephalad
    b. Anterior   d. Posterior

48. A _____ is a hollow space containing body organs.
    a. tissue   c. system
    b. organ   d. cavity

49. _____ means pertaining to both sides.
    a. Ambilateral   c. Unilateral
    b. Bilateral   d. Lateral

50. Pertaining to the groin is called:
    a. inferior   c. internal
    b. inguinal   d. organic

THE ORGANIZATION OF THE BODY
CHAPTER 2
POST TEST B

ANSWER KEY:

1.	E	26.	abd
2.	L	27.	anatomy and physiology
3.	P	28.	anterior-posterior
4.	H	29.	lat
5.	U	30.	CV
6.	A	31.	central nervous system
7.	N	32.	resp
8.	X	33.	GI
9.	R	34.	endoplasmic reticulum
10.	B	35.	posterior-anterior
11.	V	36.	d
12.	F	37.	a
13.	G	38.	c
14.	Y	39.	a
15.	K	40.	b
16.	M	41.	c
17.	Z	42.	a
18.	O	43.	c
19.	Q	44.	a
20.	S	45.	b
21.	C	46.	c
22.	I	47.	d
23.	D	48.	d
24.	J	49.	a
25.	W	50.	b

THE INTEGUMENTARY SYSTEM
CHAPTER 3
POST TEST A

PART I MULTIPLE CHOICE
DIRECTIONS: Select the best answer to each multiple choice
question and write the appropriate letter on the answer sheet.

1. The skin is essentially composed of two layers known as:
   a. epidermis and epithelium
   b. epidermis and papillary layer
   c. epidermis and dermis
   d. epidermis and reticular layer

2. A pigment which gives color to the skin is:
   a. keratin   c. melanoma
   b. melanin   d. corneum

3. The absence of pigment in the skin, hair, and eyes is
   called:
   a. albinism   c. acanthosis
   b. anhidrosis   d. alopecia

4. The medical term for "nail biting" is:
   a. onychitis   c. onychophagia
   b. onychomalacia   d. pachyonychia

5. Excessive flow of oil from the sebaceous glands is called:
   a. sebolite   c. hidrorrhea
   b. hidrosis   d. seborrhea

6. A physician may refer to a scar left after the healing of a
   wound as a:
   a. cicatrix   c. corn
   b. comedo   d. crust

7. The medical term for a bedsore is known as:
   a. keloid   c. papule
   b. macula   d. decubitus

8. The medical term tinea is also known as:
   a. chickenpox   c. measles
   b. ringworm   d. nevus

9. The combining form xero means:
   a. dry   c. hard
   b. yellow   d. soft

10. The word root pachy means:
    a. thin   c. soft
    b. hard   d. thick

24

11. The suffix rrhea means:
    a. bursting forth   c. to suture
    b. flow, discharge   d. condition of

12. Dermomycosis is a skin condition caused by a:
    a. bacterium   c. fungus
    b. virus   d. protozoan

13. A cancerous tumor that has black pigmentation is a:
    a. melanism   c. carcinomelanin
    b. melanoblastoma   d. melanocarcinoma

14. A physician who specializes in the study of the skin is a:
    a. dermatologist   c. dermatitist
    b. dermatology   d. dermalogist

15. The horny embryonic tissue from which the nail develops is:
    a. ecchymosis   c. eponychium
    b. erysipelas   d. eponym

16. _____ is an abnormal redness of the skin occurring
    over widespread areas of the body.
    a. Leukoderma   c. Xeroderma
    b. Erythroderma   d. Melanoderma

17. Overgrowth of scar tissue due to excessive collagen
    formation is called a/an:
    a. scab   c. acne
    b. cicatrix   d. keloid

18. The medical term icteric means:
    a. pertaining to jaundice   c. pertaining to the nail
    b. pertaining to the skin   d. pertaining to redness

19. The medical term subungual means pertaining to:
    a. above the nail   c. within the nail
    b. below the nail   d. beside the nail

20. A fungus condition of the hair is known as:
    a. trichiasis   c. trichomonas
    b. trichinosis   d. trichomycosis

21. The word root hidr means:
    a. sweat   c. sour
    b. sweet   d. soft

22. The suffix clysis means:
    a. solution   c. injection
    b. dissolve   d. to break

23. A plastic surgeon may perform a _____ to remove wrinkles.
    a. rhytidotomy   c. ryhtidoplasty
    b. rhizotomy   d. rhytidoplasty

24. An instrument used to cut the skin for grafting is a:
    a. dermatome   c. dermatophyte
    b. dermascope   d. dermatoscopy

25. A hypodermic injection would be given:
    a. within the skin   c. under the skin
    b. between the skin   d. above the skin

PART II MATCHING
DIRECTIONS: Using the answer sheet, write the letter of the definition that best matches the word.

26. cutaneous
27. dermatitis
28. dermatology
29. ecchymosis
30. excoriation
31. hypodermic
32. intradermal
33. melanoma
34. pediculosis
35. subcutaneous
36. alopecia
37. eczema
38. fissure
39. impetigo
40. jaundice

A. Pertaining to under the skin
B. Infestation with lice
C. Pertaining to the skin
D. A condition in which blood seeps into the skin causing discoloration
E. A malignant black mole
F. Inflammation of the skin
G. Abrasion of the epidermis
H. The study of the skin
I. An inflammatory skin disease of the epidermis
J. Icterus
K. A skin infection marked by vesicles or bullae
L. Pertaining to below the skin
M. Loss of hair
N. Pertaining to within the skin
O. An ulcer or crack-like sore
P. Hardened skin

PART III FILL-IN-THE-BLANK
DIRECTIONS: Using the answer sheet, write the correct abbreviation for each of the following.

41. _____ fever of unknown origin
42. _____ hypodermic
43. _____ history
44. _____ incision and drainage
45. _____ skin graft
46. _____ split thickness skin graft
47. _____ temperature
48. _____ ultraviolet
49. _____ xeroderma pigmentosum
50. _____ lateral

THE INTEGUMENTARY SYSTEM
CHAPTER 3
POST TEST A

ANSWER KEY:

1.	c	26.	C
2.	b	27.	F
3.	a	28.	H
4.	c	29.	D
5.	d	30.	G
6.	a	31.	A
7.	d	32.	N
8.	b	33.	E
9.	a	34.	B
10.	d	35.	L
11.	b	36.	M
12.	c	37.	I
13.	d	38.	O
14.	a	39.	K
15.	c	40.	J
16.	b	41.	FUO
17.	d	42.	H
18.	a	43.	Hx
19.	b	44.	I&D
20.	d	45.	SG
21.	a	46.	STSG
22.	c	47.	T
23.	d	48.	UV
24.	a	49.	XDP
25.	c	50.	lat

THE INTEGUMENTARY SYSTEM
CHAPTER 3
POST TEST B

PART I WORD PARTS
DIRECTIONS: Using the answer sheet, write the letter of the definition that best matches the word part.

1. an		A.	white
2. auto		B.	red
3. hyper		C.	jaundice
4. hypo		D.	black
5. intra		E.	process
6. acanth		F.	nail
7. actin		G.	wrinkle
8. aden		H.	skin
9. albin		I.	self
10. carcin		J.	sweat
11. caus		K.	cancer
12. derma		L.	heat
13. erythro		M.	without, lack of
14. hidr		N.	excessive
15. icter		O.	under
16. kerat		P.	pertaining to
17. melano		Q.	condition of
18. myc		R.	pain
19. onycho		S.	excision
20. rhytid		T.	within
21. -al		U.	a thorn
22. -algia		V.	ray
23. -ectomy		W.	gland
24. -ion		X.	horn
25. -ism		Y.	fungus
		Z.	incision

PART II FILL-IN-THE-BLANK
DIRECTIONS: Using the answer sheet, write the correct abbreviation or meaning for each of the following.

26. FUO		31.	SLE
27. hypodermic		32.	subcutaneous
28. Hx		33.	temperature
29. I&D		34.	ung
30. skin graft		35.	UV

DIRECTIONS: Select the best answer to each multiple choice question and write the appropriate letter on the answer sheet.

36. The _____ _____ is an intradermal test performed using a sterile, disposable multiple puncture lancet.
    a. patch test   c. Tine/Mono-Vacc
    b. Mantoux test   d. Tzank test

37. A test done on wound exudate to determine the presence of microorganisms.
    a. sweat test   c. Tzank test
    b. biopsy   d. wound culture

38. A microscopic examination of a small piece of tissue that has been surgically scraped from a pustule is:
    a. Tzank test   c. biopsy
    b. sweat test   d. wound culture

39. _____ is transmitted to humans by mammals and birds.
    a. Trichinosis   c. Histoplasmosis
    b. Toxoplasmosis   d. Blastomycosis

40. _____ is caused by the eating of infected, poorly cooked pork.
    a. Trichinosis   c. Histoplasmosis
    b. Toxoplasmosis   d. Blastomycosis

41. Small, pinpoint, purplish hemorrhagic spots on the skin are called:
    a. acne   c. petechiae
    b. leukoplakia   d. comedo

42. _____ is a severe itching.
    a. Alopecia   c. Decubitus
    b. Cicatrix   d. Pruritus

43. The separation or bursting open of a surgical wound is called:
    a. dehiscence   c. cicatrix
    b. exudate   d. pustule

44. A/An _____ is commonly called a blackhead.
    a. acne   c. comedo
    b. cicatrix   d. exudate

45. A _____ is a bedsore.
    a. decubitus   c. pruritus
    b. petechiae   d. scale

46. The scar left after the healing of a wound.
    a. scale   c. cicatrix
    b. scar   d. striae

47. _____ is also known as a ringworm.
    a. Rubella   c. Scabies
    b. Rubeola   d. Tinea

48. _____ is also known as chickenpox.
    a. Varicella   c. Scabies
    b. Rubeola   d. Rubella

49. _____ is also known as a mole.
    a. Nodule   c. Papule
    b. Nevus   d. Psoriasis

50. To pull or draw tight a surface, such as skin, is called:
    a. eschar   c. taut
    b. intertrigo   d. striae

THE INTEGUMENTARY SYSTEM
CHAPTER 3
POST TEST B

ANSWER KEY:

1.	M	26.	fever of unknown origin
2.	I	27.	H
3.	N	28.	history
4.	O	29.	incision & drainage
5.	T	30.	SG
6.	U	31.	systemic lupus erythematous
7.	V	32.	subcu; subq
8.	W	33.	T
9.	A	34.	ointment
10.	K	35.	ultraviolet
11.	L	36.	c
12.	H	37.	d
13.	B	38.	a
14.	J	39.	b
15.	C	40.	a
16.	X	41.	c
17.	D	42.	d
18.	Y	43.	a
19.	F	44.	c
20.	G	45.	a
21.	P	46.	c
22.	R	47.	d
23.	S	48.	a
24.	E	49.	b
25.	Q	50.	c

PART I MULTIPLE CHOICE
DIRECTIONS: Select the best answer to each multiple choice question and write the appropriate letter on the answer sheet.

1. The _____ is the shaft of a long bone.
   a. epiphysis   c. diaphysis
   b. periosteum   d. endosteum

2. A _____ is an air cavity within certain bones.
   a. fissure   c. meatus
   b. fossa   d. sinus

3. _____ is a process of moving a body part away from the middle.
   a. Abduction   c. Eversion
   b. Adduction   d. Inversion

4. The process of bending a limb is called:
   a. extension   c. pronation
   b. flexion   d. supination

5. The surgical puncture of a joint for removal of fluid is:
   a. arthrocentesis   c. arthroplasty
   b. arthrodesis   d. arthralgia

6. A bone forming cell is an:
   a. osteoclast   c. osteoblast
   b. osteoma   d. osteoclasis

7. A condition that results in reduction of bone mass is called:
   a. osteoporosis   c. osteonecrosis
   b. osteopenia   d. osteofibroma

8. A lateral curvature of the spine is known as:
   a. lordosis   c. scoliosis
   b. kyphosis   d. scoliotone

9. The prefix syn means:
   a. separate   c. apart
   b. joined   d. together

10. The combining form acro means:
    a. crooked   c. joint
    b. extremity   d. bone

11. The word root chondr means:
    a. cancer   c. glue
    b. clavicle   d. cartilage

12. The suffix -physis means:
    a. formation   c. repair
    b. growth   d. suture

13. The suffix -rrhexis means:
    a. rupture   c. repair
    b. suture   d. flow, discharge

14. All of the following are classified as long bones except:
    a. vertebrae   c. radius
    b. humerus   d. femur

15. All of the following are functions of the skeletal system except:
    a. hemopoiesis   c. acid-base balance
    b. shape and support d. protection

16. The membrane that forms the covering of bones except at their articular surfaces is called:
    a. endosteum   c. diaphysis
    b. periosteum   d. epiphysis

17. A very large process of the femur is a:
    a. trochanter   c. tuberosity
    b. tubercle   d. condyle

18. The process of lying with face downward is:
    a. pronation   c. flexion
    b. supination   d. extension

19. The surgical excision of a cartilage is:
    a. chondroectomy   c. chondrectomy
    b. chondrotomy   d. chondralgia

20. Surgical repair of the skull is called:
    a. craniotomy   c. craniectomy
    b. cranioplasty   d. cranioclasty

21. The medical term for the big toe is:
    a. genu valgum   c. bursa
    b. genu varum   d. hallux

22. A _____ fracture occurs at the ankle and affects both bones of the lower leg.
    a. spiral   c. transverse
    b. Pott's   d. greenstick

23. Inflammation of a joint is:
    a. arthritis   c. arthropathy
    b. osteoarthritis   d. arthrectomy

24. The medical term for the heel bone is:
    a. carpal
    b. carpopedal
    c. calcaneal
    d. coccygeal

25. The medical term for a fingerprint is:
    a. dactylic
    b. dactylogram
    c. dactylograph
    d. dactylogryposis

PART II MATCHING
DIRECTIONS: Using the answer sheet, write the letter of the definition that best matches the word.

26. arthralgia
27. arthrectomy
28. bursitis
29. carpoptosis
30. craniectomy
31. intercostal
32. kyphosis
33. lumbar
34. olecranal
35. pedal
36. phalangeal
37. scapular
38. genu valgum
39. sprain
40. xiphoid

A. Pertaining to the elbow
B. Resembling a sword
C. Twisting of a joint that causes pain and disability
D. Pain in a joint
E. Pertaining to the foot
F. Knock-knee
G. Bowleg
H. Pertaining to the bones of the fingers and the toes
I. Surgical excision of a joint
J. Inflammation of a bursa
K. Surgical excision of a portion of the skull
L. Pertaining to between the ribs
M. Pertaining to the shoulder blade
N. Pertaining to the loins
O. Humpback
P. Wrist drop

PART III FILL-IN-THE-BLANK
DIRECTIONS: Using the answer sheet, write the correct abbreviation for each of the following:

41. _____ temporomandibular joint
42. _____ calcium
43. _____ degenerative joint disease
44. _____ fracture
45. _____ traction
46. _____ juvenile rheumatoid arthritis
47. _____ joint
48. _____ knee jerk
49. _____ ligament
50. _____ partial weight bearing

THE SKELETAL SYSTEM
CHAPTER 4
POST TEST A

ANSWER KEY:

1.	c	26.	D
2.	d	27.	I
3.	a	28.	J
4.	b	29.	P
5.	a	30.	K
6.	c	31.	L
7.	a	32.	O
8.	c	33.	N
9.	d	34.	A
10.	b	35.	E
11.	d	36.	H
12.	b	37.	M
13.	a	38.	F
14.	a	39.	C
15.	c	40.	B
16.	b	41.	TMJ
17.	a	42.	Ca
18.	a	43.	DJD
19.	c	44.	Fx
20.	b	45.	Tx
21.	d	46.	JRA
22.	b	47.	jt
23.	a	48.	KJ
24.	c	49.	lig
25.	b	50.	PWB

THE SKELETAL SYSTEM
CHAPTER 4
POST TEST B

PART I WORD PARTS
DIRECTIONS: Using the answer sheet, write the letter of the definition that best matches the word part.

1. epi
2. inter
3. meta
4. peri
5. sub
6. sym
7. arthr
8. burs
9. carpo
10. chondro
11. cleido
12. coccygo
13. costo
14. cranio
15. kyph
16. lord
17. osteo
18. -desis
19. -itis
20. -malacia
21. -oma
22. -penia
23. -pexy
24. -plasty
25. -poiesis

A. surgical repair
B. joint
C. wrist
D. clavicle
E. a hump
F. bone
G. tumor
H. upon
I. together
J. binding
K. lack of
L. between
M. cartilage
N. tailbone
O. inflammation
P. fixation
Q. beyond
R. softening
S. hardening
T. formation
U. around
V. under, beneath
W. a pouch
X. rib
Y. bending
Z. skull

PART II FILL-IN-THE-BLANK
DIRECTIONS: Using the answer sheet, write the correct abbreviation or meaning for each of the following.

26. CDH
27. DJD
28. long leg cast
29. osteoarthritis
30. PEMFs

31. rheumatoid arthritis
32. SPECT
33. thoracic vertebra, first
34. temporomandibular joint
35. Tx

PART III MULTIPLE CHOICE
DIRECTIONS: Select the best answer to each multiple choice question and write the appropriate letter on the answer sheet.

36. Which bone is not located in the upper extremity?
    a. clavicle   c. radius
    b. humerus   d. femur

37. The medical term for knock-knee is:
    a. genu valgum   c. hallux
    b. genu varum   d. genu varium

38. Abnormal anterior curvature of the spine is called:
    a. kyphosis   c. scoliosis
    b. lordosis   d. lumbosis

39. The _____ is the shaft of a long bone.
    a. epiphysis   c. periosteum
    b. diaphysis   d. endosteum

40. An opening in the bone for blood vessels, ligaments, and nerves is called:
    a. fissure   c. foramen
    b. sinus   d. tubercle

41. _____ is the process of bending a limb.
    a. Abduction   c. Extension
    b. Eversion   d. Flexion

42. _____ is the process of lying with the face upward.
    a. Pronation   c. Protraction
    b. Supination   d. Retraction

43. _____ is an open fracture.
    a. Comminuted   c. Compound
    b. Spiral   d. Pathologic

44. _____ is also known as pes planus.
    a. Flatfoot   c. Knock-knee
    b. Clawfoot   d. Bowleg

45. The bones of the wrist are called:
    a. carpals   c. tarsals
    b. metacarpals   d. metatarsals

46. _____ is a diagnostic examination of a joint where air, followed by a radiopaque contrast medium, is injected into the joint space, x-rays are taken, and internal injuries of the meniscus, cartilage and ligaments may be seen, if present.
    a. Arthroscopy   c. Arthrography
    b. Goniometry   d. Thermography

47. The process of recording heat patterns of the body's surface is called:
   a. arthrography   c. goniometry
   b. arthroscopy   d. thermography

48. _____ is increased in gout, arthritis, multiple myeloma, and rheumatism.
   a. Calcium   c. Uric acid
   b. Phosphorus   d. Alkaline phosphatase

49. _____ level of the blood may be increased in osteoporosis and fracture healing.
   a. Sodium   c. Uric acid
   b. Phosphorus   d. Alkaline phosphatase

50. _____ is/are present in a variety of immunologic diseases.
   a. Alkaline phosphatase c. Antinuclear antibodies
   b. C-Reactive protein   d. Uric acid

THE SKELETAL SYSTEM
CHAPTER 4
POST TEST B

ANSWER KEY:

1.	H	26.	congenital dislocation of hip
2.	L	27.	degenerative joint disease
3.	Q	28.	LLC
4.	U	29.	OA
5.	V	30.	pulsing electromagnetic fields
6.	I	31.	RA
7.	B	32.	single photon emission
8.	W		computed tomography
9.	C	33.	T-1
10.	M	34.	TMJ
11.	D	35.	Traction
12.	N	36.	d
13.	X	37.	a
14.	Z	38.	b
15.	E	39.	b
16.	Y	40.	c
17.	F	41.	d
18.	J	42.	b
19.	O	43.	c
20.	R	44.	a
21.	G	45.	a
22.	K	46.	c
23.	P	47.	d
24.	A	48.	c
25.	T	49.	b
		50.	c

THE MUSCULAR SYSTEM
CHAPTER 5
POST TEST A

PART I MULTIPLE CHOICE
DIRECTIONS: Select the best answer to each multiple choice question and write the appropriate letter on the answer sheet.

1. A wide, thin, sheet-like tendon is known as an:
   a. apophysis
   b. aponeurology
   c. aponeurosis
   d. antagonist

2. All of the following are functions of the muscular system except:
   a. produce heat
   b. movement
   c. maintain posture
   d. hemopoiesis

3. Smooth muscle is also called:
   a. visceral
   b. striated
   c. voluntary
   d. cardiac

4. The medical term for pain in the arm is:
   a. brachialgia
   b. bradykinesia
   c. brachialis
   d. brachium

5. _____ is the faulty muscular development due to lack of nourishment.
   a. Dystonia
   b. Dystrophy
   c. Atrophy
   d. Atomic

6. The surgical repair of a fascia is:
   a. faciodesis
   b. fascitis
   c. fasciectomy
   d. fascioplasty

7. The point of attachment of a muscle to the part that it moves is called:
   a. insertion
   b. origin
   c. levator
   d. prime mover

8. _____ means pertaining to having equal measure.
   a. Isotonic
   b. Isometric
   c. Isomer
   d. Isomeric

9. An abnormal anterior curve of the spine is called:
   a. scoliosis
   b. kyphosis
   c. torticollis
   d. lordosis

10. _____ is the destruction of muscle tissue.
    a. Myolysis
    b. Myoclonia
    c. Myogenesis
    d. Myomalacia

11. A malignant tumor derived from muscle tissue is:
    a. myoma   c. myosarcoma
    b. myosclerosis   d. myospasm

12. A condition in which there is an abnormal darkening of muscle tissue is:
    a. myoparesis   c. myorrhaphy
    b. myomelanosis   d. myorrhexis

13. The combining form quadri means:
    a. four   c. three
    b. two   d. six

14. The suffix -desis means:
    a. surgical repair   c. binding
    b. excision   d. incision

15. The prefix intra means:
    a. outside   c. between
    b. within   d. together

16. A tumor of striated muscle tissue is:
    a. rhacoma   c. rabdomyoma
    b. rheumatism   d. rhabdomyoma

17. A plasma membrane surrounding each striated muscle fiber is:
    a. sarcoblast   c. sarcoma
    b. sarcolemma   d. sarcolysis

18. The medical term for pain in a tendon is:
    a. tenodesis   c. tenorrhaphy
    b. tenotomy   d. tenodynia

19. _____ is a muscle having three heads with a single insertion.
    a. Triceps   c. Quadriceps
    b. Biceps   d. Uniceps

20. The surgical excision of a limb, part, or other appendage is:
    a. contracture   c. amputation
    b. suspension   d. stricture

21. The medical term for a lack of muscle tone is:
    a. fatigue   c. rigor mortis
    b. flaccid   d. pallor

22. Muscles make up approximately _____ percent of a person's body weight.
    a. 46   c. 42
    b. 38   d. 32

23. The prefix apo means:
    a. lack of
    b. away from
    c. toward
    d. separation

24. The suffix -malacia means:
    a. hardening
    b. softening
    c. resembling
    d. forming

25. The _____ is a partition that separates the chest and abdominal cavities.
    a. phrenic
    b. fascia
    c. diaphragm
    d. sarcolemma

PART II MATCHING

DIRECTIONS: Using the answer sheet, write the letter of the definition that best matches the word.

26. antagonist
27. bradykinesia
28. intramuscular
29. levator
30. myasthenia
31. myomalacia
32. myorrhaphy
33. polyplegia
34. synergetic
35. tenotomy
36. voluntary
37. flaccid
38. acetylcholine
39. fatigue
40. origin

A. The beginning of anything
B. Pertaining to under the control of one's will
C. A state of tiredness occurring in a muscle as a result of repeated contractions
D. A muscle that counteracts the action of another muscle
E. Surgical incision of a tendon
F. Lack of muscle tone
G. It acts on the membrane of the muscle fiber causing generation of impulses
H. Slowness of motion
I. A muscle that raises a part
J. Pertaining to within a muscle
K. Suture of a muscle wound
L. Muscle weakness
M. Muscle strength
N. Softening of muscle tissue
O. Paralysis affecting many muscles
P. Pertaining to certain muscles that work together

PART III FILL-IN-THE-BLANK

DIRECTIONS: Using the answer sheet, write the correct abbreviation for each of the following.

41. _____ full range of motion
42. _____ limitation or loss of motion
43. _____ musculoskeletal
44. _____ physical medicine
45. _____ physical medicine and rehabilitation
46. _____ range of motion
47. _____ shoulder
48. _____ weight
49. _____ total body weight
50. _____ height

ANSWER KEY:

1.	c	26.	D
2.	d	27.	H
3.	a	28.	J
4.	a	29.	I
5.	b	30.	L
6.	d	31.	N
7.	a	32.	K
8.	b	33.	O
9.	d	34.	P
10.	a	35.	E
11.	c	36.	B
12.	b	37.	F
13.	a	38.	G
14.	c	39.	C
15.	b	40.	A
16.	d	41.	FROM
17.	b	42.	LOM
18.	d	43.	MS
19.	a	44.	PM
20.	c	45.	PMR
21.	b	46.	ROM
22.	c	47.	sh
23.	d	48.	Wt
24.	b	49.	TBW
25.	c	50.	Ht

THE MUSCULAR SYSTEM
CHAPTER 5
POST TEST B

PART I WORD PARTS
DIRECTIONS: Using the answer sheet, write the letter of the definition that best matches the word part.

1. apo
2. brady
3. con
4. dys
5. poly
6. tri
7. brachi
8. cleido
9. dactylo
10. erget
11. fascio
12. myo
13. rhabdo
14. sarco
15. sterno
16. teno
17. torti
18. -asthenia
19. -ceps
20. -desis
21. -kinesia
22. -lysis
23. -tome
24. -rrhaphy
25. -rrhexis

A. three
B. clavicle
C. work
D. muscle
E. slow
F. rupture
G. weakness
H. head
I. binding
J. separation
K. suture
L. motion
M. many
N. rod
O. with
P. a band
Q. twisted
R. sternum
S. sternum
T. difficult
U. instrument to cut
V. flesh
W. incision
X. arm
Y. finger or toe
Z. tendon

PART II FILL-IN-THE-BLANK
DIRECTIONS: Using the answer sheet, write the correct abbreviation or meaning for each of the following.

26. calcium
27. DTR's
28. electromyography
29. FROM
30. loss of motion

31. MS
32. range of motion
33. sh
34. triceps jerk
35. Wt

PART III MULTIPLE CHOICE

DIRECTIONS: Select the best answer to each multiple choice question and write the appropriate letter on the answer sheet.

36. A term used to describe the muscles immediately surrounding the shoulder joint is:
    a. torticollis
    b. aponeurosis
    c. rotator cuff
    d. levator

37. A protein found in muscle cells is called:
    a. acetylcholine
    b. dystrophin
    c. myotrophin
    d. lactic dehydrogenase

38. Movement of each joint through its full range of motion is what type of exercise?
    a. active
    b. isometric
    c. passive
    d. range of motion

39. _____ is the treatment of choice for soft tissue injuries and muscle injuries.
    a. Cryotherapy
    b. Massage
    c. Thermotherapy
    d. Hydrotherapy

40. The _____ position is where the body is erect, head facing forward, arms by the sides with palms to the front.
    a. Fowler's
    b. Sims'
    c. Anatomical
    d. Supine

41. A band of fibrous connective tissue serving for the attachment of muscles to bones.
    a. fascia
    b. tendon
    c. ligament
    d. bursa

42. The medical term for muscle weakness is:
    a. myalgia
    b. myasthenia
    c. myoid
    d. myomalacia

43. A malignant tumor derived from muscle tissue is called:
    a. myoma
    b. rhabdomyoma
    c. myosarcoma
    d. sarcolemma

44. What is pertaining to certain muscles that work together?
    a. antagonist
    b. prime mover
    c. extrinsic
    d. synergetic

45. The medical term for suture of a tendon is:
    a. tenorrhaphy
    b. tenotomy
    c. tenodynia
    d. tenodesis

46. A diagnostic test to help diagnose Duchenne's muscular dystrophy before symptoms appear is:
    a. creatine phosphokinase
    b. aldolase blood test
    c. calcium blood test
    d. muscle biopsy

47. A test to measure electrical activity across muscle membranes by means of electrodes that are attached to a needle which is inserted into the muscle is:
    a. muscle biopsy
    b. lactic dehydrogenase
    c. creatine phosphokinase
    d. electromyography

48. This test is also called aspartate transaminase.
    a. lactic dehydrogenase
    b. serum glutamic oxaloacetic transaminase
    c. serum glutamic pyruvic transaminase
    d. creatine phosphokinase

49. This test is also called alanine aminotransferase.
    a. lactic dehydrogenase
    b. serum glutamic oxaloacetic transaminase
    c. serum glutamic pyruvic transaminase
    d. creatine phosphokinase

50. A/An _____ is where a small piece of muscle tissue is excised and then stained for microscopic examination.
    a. muscle biopsy   c. bone biopsy
    b. electromyography   d. electrocardiography

THE MUSCULAR SYSTEM
CHAPTER 5
POST TEST B

1. J
2. E
3. O
4. S
5. M
6. A
7. X
8. B
9. Y
10. C
11. P
12. D
13. N
14. V
15. R
16. Z
17. Q
18. G
19. H
20. I
21. L
22. T
23. U
24. K
25. F

26. Ca
27. deep tendon reflexes
28. EMG
29. full range of motion
30. LOM
31. musculoskeletal
32. ROM
33. shoulder
34. TJ
35. weight
36. c
37. b
38. d
39. a
40. c
41. b
42. b
43. c
44. d
45. a
46. b
47. d
48. b
49. c
50. a

THE DIGESTIVE SYSTEM
CHAPTER 6
POST TEST A

PART I MULTIPLE CHOICE
DIRECTIONS: Select the best answer to each multiple choice question and write the appropriate letter on the answer sheet.

1. All of the following are functions of the digestive system except:
   a. absorption   c. digestion
   b. locomotion   d. elimination

2. A small mass of masticated food ready to be swallowed is:
   a. bolus   c. anabolism
   b. chyme   d. catabolism

3. The _____ is the first portion of the small intestine.
   a. ileum   c. cecum
   b. jejunum   d. duodenum

4. The _____ is the largest glandular organ in the body.
   a. pancreas   c. liver
   b. gallbladder   d. heart

5. The prefix post means:
   a. before   c. difficult
   b. after   d. below

6. The combining form ano means:
   a. anus   c. up
   b. appetite   d. starch

7. The word root enter means:
   a. stomach   c. within
   b. gallbladder   d. intestine

8. The suffix -ase means:
   a. pertaining to   c. condition of
   b. enzyme   d. starch

9. The medical term for pertaining to the cheek is:
   a. buccal   c. celiac
   b. biliary   d. colonic

10. _____ is an examination of the upper portion of the colon.
    a. Colonoscope   c. Colonoscopy
    b. Proctoscopy   d. Proctoscope

11. The creation of a new opening into the colon is called:
    a. colostomy   c. colorrhaphy
    b. colotomy   d. colonic

12. The medical term for a toothache is:
    a. dentoid   c. dentalgia
    b. denticle   d. dentibuccal

13. The medical term for indigestion is:
    a. dyspepsia   c. stomatitis
    b. dysphagia   d. ascites

14. The study of the stomach and the intestine is:
    a. gastrology   c. gastroenterology
    b. enterology   d. enterogastrology

15. _____ is inflammation of the liver.
    a. Hepatoma   c. Nephroma
    b. Nephritis   d. Hepatitis

16. A condition in which the colon is extremely enlarged is:
    a. diverticulitis   c. enteritis
    b. megacolon   d. microcolon

17. The surgical incision into the abdomen is:
    a. ileostomy   c. herniotomy
    b. vagotomy   d. laparotomy

18. Inflammation of the pancreas is:
    a. pancreasitis   c. pancreatin
    b. pancreatitis   d. pancreatic

19. A physician who specializes in the study of the anus and the rectum is called a:
    a. proctalgia   c. proctologist
    b. proctology   d. proctoplasty

20. A hernia of part of the rectum into the vagina is called:
    a. rectocele   c. rectostenosis
    b. rectolingual   d. rectouretheral

21. Inflammation of the salivary gland is known as:
    a. saladenitis   c. sialaden
    b. sialadenitis   d. sialoangitis

22. An accumulation of serous fluid in the peritoneal cavity is:
    a. melena   c. eructation
    b. deglutition   d. ascites

23. The medical term for vomiting is:
    a. dysentery   c. emesis
    b. eructation   d. halitosis

24. _____ means pertaining to after meals.
   a. Postocular   c. Postictal
   b. Postfebrile   d. Postprandial

25. All of the following medical terms are spelled correctly
   except:
   a. vagotomy   c. peristalsis
   b. verinform   d. enteroclysis

PART II MATCHING
DIRECTIONS: Using the answer sheet, write the letter of the
definition that best matches the word.

26. amylase   A. Difficulty in swallowing
27. anorexia   B. Inflammation of the liver
28. cholecystectomy   C. Vomiting of blood
29. colostomy   D. Pertaining to the tongue
30. dysphagia   E. An enzyme that breaks down
31. hematemesis   starch
32. hepatitis   F. Surgical excision of the
33. lingual   gallbladder
34. peptic   G. Difficulty in digestion
35. postprandial   H. Pertaining to the gatekeeper
36. pyloric   I. Lack of appetite
37. ascites   J. Bad breath
38. emesis   K. The creation of a new opening
39. flatus   into the colon
40. halitosis   L. Pertaining to gastric
                            digestion
                         M. Gas in the stomach/intestines
                         N. An accumulation of serous fluid
                            in the peritoneal cavity
                         O. Vomiting
                         P. Pertaining to after a meal

PART III FILL-IN-THE-BLANK
DIRECTIONS: Using the answer sheet, write the correct
abbreviation for each of the following.

41. _____ barium enema
42. _____ bowel movement
43. _____ bathroom privileges
44. _____ bowel sounds
45. _____ cholesterol
46. _____ carbohydrate
47. _____ food (cibus)
48. _____ chronic ulcerative colitis
49. _____ Escherichia coli
50. _____ gallbladder

THE DIGESTIVE SYSTEM
CHAPTER 6
POST TEST A

ANSWER KEY:

1.	b	26.	E
2.	a	27.	I
3.	d	28.	F
4.	c	29.	K
5.	b	30.	A
6.	a	31.	C
7.	d	32.	B
8.	b	33.	D
9.	a	34.	L
10.	c	35.	P
11.	a	36.	H
12.	c	37.	N
13.	a	38.	O
14.	c	39.	M
15.	d	40.	J
16.	b	41.	Ba E
17.	d	42.	BM
18.	b	43.	BRP
19.	c	44.	BS
20.	a	45.	ch, chol
21.	b	46.	CHO
22.	d	47.	cib
23.	c	48.	CUC
24.	d	49.	E. coli
25.	b	50.	GB

THE DIGESTIVE SYSTEM
CHAPTER 6
POST TEST B

PART I WORD PARTS
DIRECTIONS: Using the answer sheet, write the letter of the definition that best matches the word part.

1. ana
2. cata
3. retro
4. amyl
5. ano
6. cheil
7. bucc
8. chole
9. colo
10. dent
11. entero
12. esophago
13. gastro
14. gingiv
15. glosso
16. hepato
17. ileo
18. prandi
19. procto
20. vermi
21. -emesis
22. -orexia
23. -pepsia
24. -phagia
25. -stalsis

A. lip
B. vomiting
C. colon
D. stomach
E. intestine
F. gums
G. backward
H. tongue
I. worm
J. up
K. gall, bile
L. appetite
M. down
N. to digest
O. anus
P. tooth
Q. to eat
R. starch
S. contraction
T. rectum, anus
U. cheek
V. esophagus
W. pain
X. ileum
Y. liver
Z. meal

PART II FILL-IN-THE-BLANK
DIRECTIONS: Using the answer sheet, write the correct abbreviation or meaning for each of the following.

26. a.c.
27. p.c.
28. barium enema
29. bowel movement
30. CHO
31. food
32. GB
33. nasogastric
34. NPO
35. TPN

PART III MULTIPLE CHOICE
DIRECTIONS: Select the best answer to each multiple choice
question and write the appropriate letter on the answer sheet.

36. An accumulation of serous fluid in the peritoneal cavity is:
    a. peristalsis   c. melena
    b. ascites   d. eructation

37. _____ is the twisting of the bowel upon itself that
    causes an obstruction.
    a. Paralytic ileus   c. Hernia
    b. Deglutition   d. Volvulus

38. The medical term for gas in the stomach is called:
    a. flatus   c. eructation
    b. diarrhea   d. feces

39. _____ means chewing.
    a. Melena   c. Mastication
    b. Mastcation   d. Eructation

40. The _____ is the first portion of the small intestine.
    a. ileum   c. cecum
    b. jejunum   d. duodenum

41. The _____ is the largest glandular organ in the body.
    a. pancreas   c. liver
    b. gallbladder   d. heart

42. The creation of a new opening into the colon is called:
    a. colostomy   c. colorrhaphy
    b. colotomy   d. colonic

43. The medical term for indigestion is:
    a. dyspepsia   c. stomatitis
    b. dysphagia   d. ascites

44. _____ is the surgical incision into the abdomen.
    a. Ileostomy   c. Herniotomy
    b. Vagotomy   d. Laparotomy

45. All of the following terms are spelled correctly except:
    a. vagotomy   c. peristalsis
    b. verinform   d. enteroclysis

46. Fluoroscopic examination of the esophagus, stomach, and small
    intestine.
    a. barium enema   c. cholangiography
    b. ultrasonography   d. gastrointestinal series

47. An endoscopic examination of the esophagus, stomach, and
    small intestine.
    a. cholangiography
    b. gastroduodenoesophagoscopy
    c. esophagogastroduodenoscopy
    d. gastric analysis

48. A quantitative assay test that detects heme in the stool.
    a. occult blood test   c. Hemo Quant test
    b. stool culture   d. ova and parasites test

49. X-ray examination of the common bile duct, cystic duct, and
    hepatic ducts.
    a. cholangiography   c. cholangiopancreatography
    b. cholecystography   d. ultrasonography

50. The direct visual examination of the colon via a flexible
    colonoscope.
    a. cholangiography   c. colonofiberoscopy
    b. ultrasonography   d. cholecystography

THE DIGESTIVE SYSTEM
CHAPTER 6
POST TEST B

ANSWER KEY:

1.	J	26.	before meals
2.	M	27.	after meals
3.	G	28.	BaE
4.	R	29.	BM
5.	O	30.	carbohydrate
6.	A	31.	cib
7.	U	32.	gallbladder
8.	K	33.	NG
9.	C	34.	nothing by mouth
10.	P	35.	total parenteral
11.	E		nutrition
12.	V	36.	b
13.	D	37.	d
14.	F	38.	a
15.	H	39.	c
16.	Y	40.	d
17.	X	41.	c
18.	Z	42.	a
19.	T	43.	a
20.	I	44.	d
21.	B	45.	b
22.	L	46.	d
23.	N	47.	c
24.	Q	48.	c
25.	S	49.	a
		50.	c

THE CARDIOVASCULAR SYSTEM
CHAPTER 7
POST TEST A

PART I MULTIPLE CHOICE
DIRECTIONS: Select the best answer to each multiple choice question and write the appropriate letter on the answer sheet.

1. The _____ is the inner lining of the heart.
   a. myocardium   c. pericardium
   b. endocardium   d. septum

2. The heart weighs approximately _____ grams.
   a. 400   c. 360
   b. 200   d. 300

3. All of the following are primary pulse points except:
   a. popliteal   c. brachial
   b. radial   d. carotid

4. _____ _____ is the pressure exerted by the blood on the walls of the vessels.
   a. Pulse pressure   c. Blood pressure
   b. Systolic pressure   d. Diastolic pressure

5. Blood is transported from the right and left ventricles of the heart to all body parts by the:
   a. veins   c. capillaries
   b. arteries   d. atria

6. A condition in which there is a lack of rhythm of the heart beat is:
   a. murmur   c. arrhythmia
   b. palpitation   d. fibrillation

7. A slow heartbeat is called:
   a. bradycardia   c. brachycardia
   b. tachycardia   d. murmur

8. The medical term for hardening of the arteries is:
   a. atherosclerosis   c. arteriosclerosis
   b. arteriotome   d. atheroma

9. A type of medication which increases the tone of the heart is called:
   a. vasodilator   c. cardiopathy
   b. vasotonic   d. cardiotonic

10. A condition in which a blood clot obstructs a blood vessel is known as:
    a. thrombosis   c. cyanosis
    b. embolism   d. constriction

11. The surgical excision of the inner portion of an artery is called:
    a. endarterotomy   c. endarteritis
    b. endocardium   d. endarterectomy

12. A tumor of a blood vessel is called:
    a. hemangioma   c. aneurysm
    b. hematoma   d. angionecrosis

13. An incision into a vein is known as:
    a. phlebolith   c. phlebitis
    b. phlebotomy   d. phlebectomy

14. A fast heartbeat is known as:
    a. bradycardia   c. brachycardia
    b. trachycardia   d. tachycardia

15. Tapping sounds heard during auscultation of blood pressure are called:
    a. murmur   c. bruit
    b. Korotkoff's sounds   d. systolic sounds

16. The _____ _____ is called the pacemaker.
    a. sinoatrial node   c. atrioventricular node
    b. bundle of His   d. Purkinje system

17. The _____ _____ is located in the antecubital space of the elbow.
    a. radial pulse   c. carotid pulse
    b. brachial pulse   d. femoral pulse

18. The most common site for taking a pulse is the _____ artery.
    a. carotid   c. brachial
    b. femoral   d. radial

19. A _____ is a sudden severe attack such as a blockage or rupture of a blood vessel within the brain.
    a. shock   c. infarction
    b. stroke   d. fibrillation

20. The word root angin means:
    a. vessel   c. to choke, quinsy
    b. aorta   d. to hold back

21. The combining form mano means:
    a. thick   c. thin
    b. heavy   d. light

22. The combining form phono means:
    a. sight   c. soft
    b. speech   d. sound

23. The suffix -emia means:
    a. process   c. condition of
    b. blood condition   d. formation

24. _____ is an instrument used to measure the arterial blood pressure.
    a. Stethoscope   c. Sphygmomanometer
    b. Cardioscope   d. Sphygomomanometer

25. Crushing of a blood vessel to arrest hemorrhaging is:
    a. vasotripsy   c. vasospasm
    b. vasodilator   d. vasotonic

PART II MATCHING
DIRECTIONS: Using the answer sheet, write the letter of the definition that best matches the word.

26. claudication
27. cardiologist
28. cardioptosis
29. hemangioma
30. hypertension
31. hypotension
32. phlebitis
33. lipoproteins
34. stethoscope
35. triglyceride
36. venipuncture
37. aneurysm
38. diastole
39. systole
40. murmur

A. To pierce a vein
B. A soft blowing sound
C. Fat and proteins that are bound together
D. An instrument used to listen to sounds of the heart and lungs
E. The relaxation phase of the heart cycle
F. The contractive phase of the heart cycle
G. The process of lameness
H. Inflammation of a vein
I. One who specializes in the study of the heart
J. A sac formed by a local widening of the wall of an artery or a vein
K. Low blood pressure
L. High blood pressure
M. A compound that has three molecules of fatty acids
N. Prolapse of the heart
O. Tumor of a blood vessel
P. Tumor of an artery

PART III FILL-IN-THE-BLANK
DIRECTIONS: Using the answer sheet, write the correct abbreviation for each of the following.

41. _____ acute myocardial infarction
42. _____ blood pressure
43. _____ coronary artery disease
44. _____ cardiac output
45. _____ congestive heart failure
46. _____ electrocardiogram
47. _____ high density lipoprotein
48. _____ heart and lungs
49. _____ mitral stenosis
50. _____ premature ventricular contractions

THE CARDIOVASCULAR SYSTEM
CHAPTER 7
POST TEST A

ANSWER KEY:

1.	b	26.	G
2.	d	27.	I
3.	a	28.	N
4.	c	29.	O
5.	b	30.	L
6.	c	31.	K
7.	a	32.	H
8.	c	33.	C
9.	d	34.	D
10.	b	35.	M
11.	d	36.	A
12.	a	37.	J
13.	b	38.	E
14.	d	39.	F
15.	b	40.	B
16.	a	41.	AMI
17.	b	42.	BP
18.	d	43.	CAD
19.	b	44.	CO
20.	c	45.	CHF
21.	c	46.	ECG, EKG
22.	d	47.	HDL
23.	b	48.	H&L
24.	c	49.	MS
25.	a	50.	PVCs

THE CARDIOVASCULAR SYSTEM
CHAPTER 7
POST TEST B

PART I WORD PARTS
DIRECTIONS: Using the answer sheet, write the letter of the definition that best matches the word part.

1. brady
2. hyper
3. hypo
4. angi
5. arterio
6. athero
7. cardio
8. cyan
9. mano
10. phlebo
11. phono
12. scler
13. sphygmo
14. stetho
15. thromb
16. vector
17. tachy
18. -blast
19. -clysis
20. -emia
21. -graph
22. -meter
23. -scope
24. -systole
25. -pathy

A. heart
B. dark blue
C. vein
D. hardening
E. pulse
F. a carrier
G. fast
H. slow
I. immature cell
J. deficient, below
K. thin
L. chest
M. blood condition
N. vessel
O. to write
P. instrument to measure
Q. instrument
R. excessive, above
S. sound
T. fatty substance
U. contraction
V. disease
W. artery
X. incision
Y. injection
Z. clot of blood

PART II FILL-IN-THE-BLANK
DIRECTIONS: Using the answer sheet, write the correct abbreviation or meaning for each of the following.

26. atrioventricular
27. BP
28. CAD
29. electrocardiogram
30. HDL

31. myocardial infarction
32. MVP
33. PMI
34. sinoatrial
35. TPA

PART III MULTIPLE CHOICE
DIRECTIONS: Select the best answer to each multiple choice question and write the appropriate letter on the answer sheet.

36. _____ is a waxy, fat-like substance in the bloodstream of all animals.
    a. Carbohydrate   c. Lipoprotein
    b. Cholesterol   d. Tissue plasminogen

37. To gather an organ and make it ready for transplantation is:
    a. bruit   c. harvest
    b. anastomosis   d. flutter

38. The _____ is the inner lining of the heart.
    a. myocardium   c. pericardium
    b. endocardium   d. septum

39. The heart weighs approximately _____ grams.
    a. 400   c. 360
    b. 200   d. 300

40. A slow heartbeat is called:
    a. bradycardia   c. brachycardia
    b. tachycardia   d. murmur

41. A condition in which a blood clot obstructs a blood vessel is known as:
    a. embolism   c. cyanosis
    b. vasoconstriction   d. constriction

42. An incision into a vein is called:
    a. phlebolith   c. phlebitis
    b. phlebotomy   d. phlebectomy

43. A fast heartbeat is called:
    a. bradycardia   c. brachycardia
    b. trachycardia   d. tachycardia

44. The _____ _____ is located in the antecubital space of the elbow.
    a. radial pulse   c. carotid pulse
    b. brachial pulse   d. femoral pulse

45. _____ is an instrument used to measure the arterial blood pressure.
    a. Stethoscope   c. Sphygmomanometer
    b. Cardioscope   d. Sphygomomanometer

46. A method of recording a patient's ECG for 24 hours is:
    a. stress test   c. ultrasonography
    b. Holter monitor   d. angiography

47. A test used to determine the size and shape of arteries and veins of organs and tissues is:
    a. electrophysiology   c. angiogram
    b. stress test   d. cholesterol

48. The x-ray recording of a blood vessel after the injection of a radiopaque substance is:
    a. angiogram   c. stress test
    b. angiography   d. cardiac catheterization

49. _____ is a cardiac procedure that maps the electrical activity of the heart from within the heart itself.
    a. Electrocardiogram   c. Electrophysiology
    b. Electrocardiomyogram   D. Cardiac catheterization

50. Blood test performed to determine cardiac damage in an acute myocardial infarction is:
    a. cardiac enzymes   c. triglycerides
    b. cholesterol   d. angiogram

THE CARDIOVASCULAR SYSTEM
CHAPTER 7
POST TEST B

ANSWER KEY:

1.	H	26.	AV
2.	R	27.	blood pressure
3.	J	28.	coronary artery disease
4.	N	29.	ECG, EKG
5.	W	30.	high density lipoprotein
6.	T	31.	MI
7.	A	32.	mitral valve prolapse
8.	B	33.	point of maximum impulse
9.	K	34.	SA
10.	C	35.	tissue plasminogen activator
11.	S	36.	b
12.	D	37.	c
13.	E	38.	b
14.	L	39.	d
15.	Z	40.	a
16.	F	41.	a
17.	G	42.	b
18.	I	43.	d
19.	Y	44.	b
20.	M	45.	c
21.	O	46.	b
22.	P	47.	c
23.	Q	48.	b
24.	U	49.	c
25.	V	50.	a

BLOOD AND THE LYMPHATIC SYSTEM
CHAPTER 8
POST TEST A

PART I MULTIPLE CHOICE
DIRECTIONS: Select the best answer to each multiple choice
question and write the appropriate letter on the answer sheet.

1. Which of the following is not a function of the lymphatic
   system?
   a. transports proteins and fluids
   b. protects the body against pathogens
   c. produces thrombocytes
   d. serves as a pathway for the absorption of fats

2. The life span of an erythrocyte is:
   a. 80-120 days   c. 70-102 days
   b. 90-110 days   d. 120-160 days

3. All of the following are true statements about RBCs except:
   a. they are doughnut shaped cells
   b. they transport oxygen and carbon dioxide
   c. they are formed in the red bone marrow
   d. they are disk-shaped cells

4. The fluid part of the blood is called:
   a. serum   c. lymph
   b. plasma   d. hemoglobin

5. A protein substance that is produced in the body in response
   to an invading foreign substance is called:
   a. antigen   c. platelet
   b. phagocyte   d. antibody

6. The medical term for a lack of red blood cells is:
   a. erythropoiesis   c. erythrocytosis
   b. erythropenia   d. erythropathy

7. _____ is the iron containing pigment of red blood cells.
   a. Globulin   c. Hemoglobin
   b. Prothrombin   d. Corpuscle

8. Excessive bleeding, bursting forth of blood is called:
   a. hemorrhage   c. hemostasis
   b. hemophilia   d. hemophobia

9. Excessive amounts of sugar in the blood is called:
   a. hypoglycemia   c. hypercalcemia
   b. hypercapnia   d. hyperglycemia

10. _____ is the removal of WBCs from the circulation.
    a. Leukemia   c. Leukopheresis
    b. Leukocytopenia   d. Leukocyte

11. Inflammation of the lymph glands is called:
    a. lymphadenitis   c. lymphangitis
    b. lymphadenotomy   d. lymphadenia

12. An abnormally large erythrocyte is called:
    a. monocyte   c. microcyte
    b. macrocyte   d. phagocyte

13. A medical condition in which there are too many RBCs is:
    a. anemia   c. polycythemia
    b. leukemia   d. septicemia

14. A _____ is one who specializes in the study of serum.
    a. serology   c. pathologist
    b. serologist   d. pathology

15. The prefix mono means:
    a. one   c. two
    b. many   d. double

16. The combining form leuko means:
    a. yellow   c. white
    b. blue   d. red

17. The suffix -crit means:
    a. to separate   c. loosen
    b. destruction   d. protein

18. The formation of a blood clot is called:
    a. thrombocyte   c. thrombosis
    b. thrombogenic   d. thrombolysis

19. The medical term for a tumor of the thymus is:
    a. thymitis   c. thymoma
    b. thymocyte   d. thrombosis

20. A blood enzyme which causes clotting by forming fibrin is:
    a. thromboplastin   c. heparin
    b. fibrinogen   d. thrombin

21. All of the following are types of leukocytes except:
    a. neutrophils   c. reticulocytes
    b. eosinophils   d. lymphocytes

22. _____ plays an important role in the clotting process.
    a. Thrombocytes   c. Leukocytes
    b. Erythrocytes   d. Lymphocytes

23. An agent that works against the formation of blood clots is:
    a. antibody   c. antigen
    b. anticoagulant   d. antihemorrhagic

24. An immature red blood cell is called:
    a. eosinophil   c. erythroblast
    b. erythrocyte   d. erythroclast

25. _____ is the engulfing and eating of bacteria.
    a. Sideropenia   c. Thalassemia
    b. Phagocytosis   d. Thrombogenic

PART II MATCHING
DIRECTIONS: Using the answer sheet, write the letter of the definition that best matches the word.

26. agglutination	A. A blood cell
27. allergy	B. Surgical excision of a blood clot
28. embolus	
29. immunoglobulin	C. A hormone that stimulates the production of RBCs
30. hematocele	
31. hematoma	D. A clear, colorless, alkaline fluid
32. hemolysis	
33. hemopoiesis	E. The process of clumping together
34. hemostasis	
35. hypoglycemia	F. A substance that inhibits blood clotting
36. thrombectomy	
37. corpuscle	G. Individual hypersensitivity to a substance
38. heparin	
39. lymph	H. The destruction of RBCs
40. erythropoietin	I. A blood clot carried in the bloodstream
	J. A condition of deficient amounts of sugar in the blood
	K. A blood protein capable of acting as an antibody
	L. The control of bleeding
	M. To increase the flow of blood
	N. A blood cyst
	O. A blood tumor
	P. Formation of blood cells

PART III FILL-IN-THE-BLANK
DIRECTIONS: Using the answer sheet, write the correct abbreviation for each of the following.

41. _____ blood group
42. _____ acquired immunodeficiency syndrome
43. _____ acute lymphoblastic leukemia
44. _____ blood alcohol concentration
45. _____ body systems isolation
46. _____ complete blood count
47. _____ hemoglobin
48. _____ hematocrit
49. _____ red blood cell
50. _____ Rhesus (factor)

BLOOD AND THE LYMPHATIC SYSTEM
CHAPTER 8
POST TEST A

ANSWER KEY:

1.	c	26.	E
2.	a	27.	G
3.	d	28.	I
4.	b	29.	K
5.	d	30.	N
6.	b	31.	O
7.	c	32.	H
8.	a	33.	P
9.	d	34.	L
10.	c	35.	J
11.	a	36.	B
12.	b	37.	A
13.	c	38.	F
14.	b	39.	D
15.	a	40.	C
16.	c	41.	ABO
17.	a	42.	AIDS
18.	b	43.	ALL
19.	c	44.	BAC
20.	d	45.	BSI
21.	c	46.	CBC
22.	a	47.	Hb, Hgb
23.	b	48.	HCT
24.	c	49.	RBC
25.	b	50.	Rh

BLOOD AND THE LYMPHATIC SYSTEM
CHAPTER 8
POST TEST B

PART I WORD PARTS
DIRECTIONS: Using the answer sheet, write the letter of the definition that best matches the word part.

1.	pan	A.	base
2.	mono	B.	red
3.	agglutinat	C.	blood
4.	aniso	D.	eat, engulf
5.	baso	E.	whey, serum
6.	coagul	F.	work
7.	eosino	G.	all
8.	erythro	H.	lack of
9.	granulo	I.	attraction
10.	hemato	J.	unequal
11.	leuko	K.	little grain
12.	phago	L.	fear
13.	reticulo	M.	one
14.	sero	N.	formation
15.	sidero	O.	bursting forth
16.	thrombo	P.	clumping
17.	-crit	Q.	white
18.	-ergy	R.	protein
19.	-globin	S.	removal
20.	-penia	T.	to clot
21.	-pheresis	U.	clot
22.	-philia	V.	to separate
23.	-phobia	W.	rose colored
24.	-poiesis	X.	flow
25.	-rrhage	Y.	iron
		Z.	net

PART II FILL-IN-THE-BLANK
DIRECTIONS: Using the answer sheet, write the correct abbreviation or meaning for each of the following.

26.	antihemophilic factor	31.	pneumocystis pneumonia
27.	ARC	32.	PT
28.	EBV	33.	partial thromboplastin time
29.	hemoglobin	34.	RIA
30.	hematocrit	35.	WBC

PART III MULTIPLE CHOICE

DIRECTIONS: Select the best answer to each multiple choice question and write the appropriate letter on the answer sheet.

36. _____ is a hormone that stimulates the production of red blood cells.
    a. Fibrin
    b. Heparin
    c. Erythropoietin
    d. Erythropoieten

37. A blood protein capable of acting as an antibody is:
    a. immunoglobulin
    b. thromboglobulin
    c. globulin
    d. hemoglobulin

38. _____ is the fluid part of the blood.
    a. Lymph
    b. Plasma
    c. Serum
    d. Fibrin

39. A blood test performed to identify antigen-antibody reactions is:
    a. sedimentation rate
    b. hematocrit
    c. immunoglobulins
    d. antinuclear antibodies

40. This blood test includes a hematocrit, hemoglobin, red and white blood cell count, and differential:
    a. blood typing
    b. sedimentation rate
    c. CBC
    d. Hb, Hgb

41. A blood test performed on whole blood to determine the percentage of RBCs in the total blood volume is:
    a. RBC
    b. WBC
    c. Hct
    d. PTT

42. A blood test to determine the number of leukocytes present is called:
    a. RBC
    b. WBC
    c. Hct
    d. PTT

43. A puncture of the ear lobe or forearm to determine the time required for blood to stop flowing is:
    a. bleeding time
    b. platelet count
    c. prothrombin time
    d. PTT

44. The life span of an erythrocyte is:
    a. 80-120 days
    b. 90-110 days
    c. 70-102 days
    d. 120-160 days

45. _____ is the iron containing pigment of RBCs.
    a. Globulin
    b. Prothrombin
    c. Hemoglobin
    d. Corpuscle

46. All of the following are types of WBCs except:
    a. neutrophils   c. reticulocytes
    b. eosinophils   d. lymphocytes

47. An immature red blood cell is called:
    a. eosinophil   c. erythroblast
    b. erythrocyte   d. erythroclast

48. A condition in which there is a lack of RBCs is called:
    a. allergy   c. antigen
    b. anemia   d. dysemia

49. A _____ is a blood tumor.
    a. hemolysis   c. hematoma
    b. hemostasis   d. hemopoiesis

50. _____ is a lack of iron in the blood.
    a. Polycythemia   c. Septicemia
    b. Sideropenia   d. Splenemia

BLOOD AND THE LYMPHATIC SYSTEM
CHAPTER 8
POST TEST B

ANSWER KEY:

1.	G	26.	AHF
2.	M	27.	AIDS related complex
3.	P	28.	Epstein-Barr virus
4.	J	29.	Hb, Hgb
5.	A	30.	Hct
6.	T	31.	PCP
7.	W	32.	prothrombin time
8.	B	33.	PTT
9.	K	34.	radioimmunoassay
10.	C	35.	white blood cell (count)
11.	Q	36.	c
12.	D	37.	a
13.	Z	38.	b
14.	E	39.	d
15.	Y	40.	c
16.	U	41.	c
17.	V	42.	b
18.	F	43.	a
19.	R	44.	a
20.	H	45.	c
21.	S	46.	c
22.	I	47.	c
23.	L	48.	b
24.	N	49.	c
25.	O	50.	b

THE RESPIRATORY SYSTEM
CHAPTER 9
POST TEST A

PART I MULTIPLE CHOICE
DIRECTIONS: Select the best answer to each multiple choice question and write the appropriate letter on the answer sheet.

1. All of the following are organs of the respiratory system except:
    a. nose
    b. pharynx
    c. lungs
    d. tonsils

2. The _____ acts as a lid to prevent aspiration of food into the trachea.
    a. glottis
    b. epiglottis
    c. cricoid
    d. hilum

3. The central portion of the thoracic cavity, between the lungs, is a space called the:
    a. mediastinum
    b. septum
    c. diaphragm
    d. bronchi

4. The air cells of the lungs are the:
    a. cilia
    b. pleura
    c. alveoli
    d. bronchi

5. The respiratory rate for an adult is ___ to ___ breaths per minute.
    a. 12-16
    b. 15-20
    c. 18-24
    d. 16-32

6. A condition in which there is a lack of the sense of smell is:
    a. anoxia
    b. aphonia
    c. apnea
    d. anosmia

7. A temporary cessation of breathing is known as:
    a. apnea
    b. dyspnea
    c. atelectasis
    d. cyanosis

8. A _____ is an instrument used to examine the bronchi.
    a. spirometer
    b. laryngoscope
    c. bronchoscope
    d. spirogram

9. The medical term for difficulty in breathing is:
    a. apnea
    b. hypoxia
    c. eupnea
    d. dyspnea

10. The medical term for spitting up of blood is:
    a. hemoptysis
    b. hemothorax
    c. epistaxis
    d. pertussis

11. _____ is the establishing of a new opening in the larynx.
   a. Laryngostenosis   c. Laryngotomy
   b. Laryngostomy   d. Laryngectomy

12. The inability to breathe unless in an upright position is:
   a. apnea   c. dyspnea
   b. eupnea   d. orthopnea

13. _____ is a condition of the lung due to the inhalation of dust.
   a. Pneumoconiosis   c. Pneumonia
   b. Pneumonitis   d. Pneumothorax

14. _____ is the surgical repair of the nose.
   a. Rhinorrhagia   c. Rhinoplasty
   b. Rhinorrhea   d. Rhinotomy

15. A _____ is an instrument used to measure the volume of respired air.
   a. spirogram   c. pulmometer
   b. respirator   d. spirometer

16. The medical term for fast breathing is:
   a. tachycardia   c. bradypnea
   b. tachypnea   d. bradycardia

17. The surgical puncture of the chest for removal of fluid is:
   a. thoracopathy   c. thoracoplasty
   b. thoracotomy   d. thoracocentesis

18. The medical term for the common cold is:
   a. croup   c. pertussis
   b. coryza   d. epistaxis

19. _____ is a condition where the lung is collapsed.
   a. Asthma   c. Atelectasis
   b. Aspiration   d. Asphyxia

20. _____ is pus in the pleural cavity.
   a. Empyema   c. Epistaxis
   b. Emphysema   d. Rhonchus

21. The medical term for whooping cough is:
   a. pleurisy   c. polyp
   b. pertussis   d. rale

22. _____ _____ is the amount of air in a single inspiration or expiration.
   a. Residual volume   c. Total capacity
   b. Vital capacity   d. Tidal volume

23. The musculomembranous wall that separates the thoracic and abdominal cavity is called:
   a. mediastinum
   b. septum
   c. diaphragm
   d. hilum

24. The word root anthrac means:
   a. cold
   b. coal
   c. dust
   d. pus

25. The suffix -phore means:
   a. bearing
   b. stroke
   c. flow
   d. pain

PART II MATCHING
DIRECTIONS: Using the answer sheet, write the letter of the definition that best matches the word.

26. anoxia	A. Surgical excision of the tonsils
27. aphonia	
28. bronchiectasis	B. Discharge from the nose
29. cyanosis	C. Good or normal breathing
30. eupnea	D. Inflammation of the larynx
31. hemothorax	E. Nosebleed
32. inhalation	F. Incision into the chest
33. laryngitis	G. Lack of oxygen
34. pharyngitis	H. Blood in the chest cavity
35. rhinoscopy	I. The process of breathing air into the lungs
36. rhinorrhea	
37. thoracotomy	J. A rhythmic cycle of breathing with an increase in respiration followed by apnea
38. tonsillectomy	
39. Cheyne-Stokes respiration	K. A lack of vocal sound
40. epistaxis	L. Dilation of the bronchi
	M. Inflammation of the pharynx
	N. Inflammation of the trachea
	O. Visual examination of the nasal passages
	P. Dark blue condition

PART III FILL-IN-THE-BLANK
DIRECTIONS: Write the correct abbreviation.

41. _____ acute respiratory disease
42. _____ cystic fibrosis
43. _____ chronic obstructive pulmonary disease
44. _____ hyaline membrane disease
45. _____ intermittent positive-pressure breathing
46. _____ oxygen
47. _____ postnasal drip
48. _____ respiration
49. _____ respiratory distress syndrome
50. _____ sudden infant death syndrome

THE RESPIRATORY SYSTEM
CHAPTER 9
POST TEST A

ANSWER KEY:

1.	d	26.	G
2.	b	27.	K
3.	a	28.	L
4.	c	29.	P
5.	b	30.	C
6.	d	31.	H
7.	a	32.	I
8.	c	33.	D
9.	d	34.	M
10.	a	35.	O
11.	b	36.	B
12.	d	37.	F
13.	a	38.	A
14.	c	39.	J
15.	d	40.	E
16.	b	41.	ARD
17.	d	42.	CF
18.	b	43.	COPD
19.	c	44.	HMD
20.	a	45.	IPPB
21.	b	46.	O_2
22.	d	47.	PND
23.	c	48.	R
24.	b	49.	RDS
25.	a	50.	SIDS

THE RESPIRATORY SYSTEM
CHAPTER 9
POST TEST B

PART I WORD PARTS
DIRECTIONS: Using the answer sheet, write the letter of the definition that best matches the word part.

1.	eu	A.	to spit
2.	aero	B.	voice
3.	alveol	C.	breathing
4.	anthrac	D.	hernia
5.	atel	E.	coal
6.	broncho	F.	pus
7.	laryngo	G.	bronchi
8.	myc	H.	fungus
9.	naso	I.	nose
10.	ortho	J.	oxygen
11.	osm	K.	good
12.	ox	L.	smell
13.	pharyng	M.	pharynx
14.	phon	N.	imperfect
15.	phras	O.	surgical puncture
16.	pneumo	P.	speech
17.	pulmo	Q.	air
18.	pyo	R.	bearing
19.	thoraco	S.	lung, air
20.	tracheo	T.	chest
21.	-cele	U.	small, hollow air sac
22.	-centesis	V.	lung
23.	-phore	W.	larynx
24.	-pnea	X.	trachea
25.	-ptysis	Y.	narrowing
		Z.	straight

PART II FILL-IN-THE-BLANK
DIRECTIONS: Using the answer sheet, write the correct abbreviation or meaning for each of the following.

26.	chest x-ray	31.	T&A
27.	ET	32.	TB
28.	MBC	33.	tidal volume
29.	postnasal drip	34.	URI
30.	shortness of breath	35.	vital capacity

PART III MULTIPLE CHOICE
DIRECTIONS: Select the best answer to each multiple choice question and write the appropriate letter on the answer sheet.

36. The medical term for the common cold is:
    a. croup   c. pertussis
    b. coryza   d. pollinosis

37. The medical term for hay fever is:
    a. croup   c. pertussis
    b. coryza   d. pollinosis

38. _____ is the process of smelling.
    a. Olfaction   c. Aspiration
    b. Inhalation   d. Oxygenation

39. _____ is the substance coughed up from the lungs.
    a. Wheeze   c. Rale
    b. Rhonchus   d. Sputum

40. A test performed on sputum to detect the presence of mycobacterium tuberculi is:
    a. antistreptolysin O   c. pulmonary function
    b. acid-fast bacilli   d. bronchoscopy

41. The visual examination of the nasal passages is:
    a. bronchoscopy   c. rhinoscopy
    b. laryngoscopy   d. nasopharyngography

42. _____ are important in determining respiratory acidosis and/or alkalosis; metabolic acidosis and/or alkalosis.
    a. Acid-fast bacilli   c. Arterial blood gases
    b. Antistreptolysin O   d. Pulmonary function tests

43. _____ is a series of tests performed to determine the diffusion of oxygen and carbon dioxide across the cell membrane in the lungs.
    a. Acid-fast bacilli   c. Arterial blood gases
    b. Antistreptolysin O   d. Pulmonary function

44. The visual examination of the larynx, trachea and bronchi via a flexible scope is called:
    a. bronchoscopy   c. nasopharyngography
    b. laryngoscopy   d. rhinoscopy

45. _____ is also called air hunger.
    a. Legionnaire's disease
    b. Cystic fibrosis
    c. Kussmaul's breathing
    d. Hyperventilation

46. The _____ acts as a lid to prevent aspiration of food
    into the trachea.
    a. glottis   c. cricoid
    b. epiglottis   d. hilum

47. A temporary cessation of breathing is known as:
    a. apnea   c. atelectasis
    b. dyspnea   d. cyanosis

48. The inability to breathe unless in an upright position is:
    a. apnea   c. dyspnea
    b. eupnea   d. orthopnea

49. The medical term for spitting up of blood is:
    a. hemoptysis   c. epistaxis
    b. hemothorax   d. pertussis

50. _____ is a condition in which the lung is collapsed.
    a. Asthma   c. Atelectasis
    b. Aspiration   d. Asphyxia

THE RESPIRATORY SYSTEM
CHAPTER 9
POST TEST B

ANSWER KEY:

1.	K	26.	CXR
2.	Q	27.	endotracheal
3.	U	28.	maximal breathing capacity
4.	E	29.	PND
5.	N	30.	SOB
6.	G	31.	tonsillectomy & adenoidectomy
7.	W	32.	tuberculosis
8.	H	33.	TV
9.	I	34.	upper respiratory infection
10.	Z	35.	VC
11.	L	36.	b
12.	J	37.	d
13.	M	38.	a
14.	B	39.	d
15.	P	40.	b
16.	S	41.	c
17.	V	42.	c
18.	F	43.	d
19.	T	44.	a
20.	X	45.	c
21.	D	46.	b
22.	O	47.	a
23.	R	48.	d
24.	C	49.	a
25.	A	50.	c

THE URINARY SYSTEM
CHAPTER 10
POST TEST A

PART I MULTIPLE CHOICE
DIRECTIONS: Select the best answer to each multiple choice question and write the appropriate letter on the answer sheet.

1. The structural and functional unit of the kidney is the:
    a. neuron   c. nephron
    b. glomerulus   d. cortex

2. The inner portion of the kidney is the:
    a. cortex   c. Bowman's capsule
    b. glomerulus   d. medulla

3. A small, triangular area near the base of the bladder is:
    a. trigone   c. pelvis
    b. meatus   d. Malpighian corpuscle

4. An average daily urinary output is approximately:
    a. 1200-1600 mL   c. 800-1200 mL
    b. 1000-1500 mL   d. 1400-1800 mL

5. A routine urinalysis may include all of the following except:
    a. physical exam   c. culture
    b. chemical exam   d. microscopic exam

6. Urine is secreted and travels through which of the following organs (give the correct order)
    a. kidneys, urethra, bladder, ureters
    b. kidneys, ureters, bladder, urethra
    c. kidneys, bladder, ureters, urethra
    d. kidneys, bladder, urethra, ureters

7. A urine that has a fruity sweet odor may indicate:
    a. diabetes insipidus   c. dehydration
    b. pyelonephritis   d. diabetes mellitus

8. A medication that decreases urine secretion is called:
    a. antidiuretic   c. antibiotic
    b. diuretic   d. antiemetic

9. The medical term for inflammation of the bladder is:
    a. cystocele   c. cystoplegia
    b. cystopyelitis   d. cystitis

10. Difficult or painful urination is called:
    a. anuria   c. enuresis
    b. dysuria   d. nocturia

11. The medical term for a kidney stone is:
    a. nephrology   c. nephroma
    b. nephritis   d. nephrolith

12. _____ is excessive urination during the night.
    a. Nocturia   c. Polyuria
    b. Oliguria   d. Pyuria

13. The inflammation of the kidney and renal pelvis is:
    a. pyelocystitis   c. nephritis
    b. pyelonephritis   d. pyelitis

14. _____ is pus in the urine.
    a. Pyuria   c. Nephremia
    b. Uremia   d. Glycosuria

15. An abnormal condition in which the body tissues contain an
    accumulation of fluid is known as:
    a. ascites   c. stricture
    b. retention   d. edema

16. The external opening of the urethra is the:
    a. medulla   c. cortex
    b. meatus   d. trigone

17. _____ means pertaining to a connection between the ureter
    and bladder.
    a. Ureterostenosis   c. Ureterovesical
    b. Ureteroplasty   d. Ureterocolostomy

18. An instrument used to measure the specific gravity of urine
    is called a/an:
    a. urinometer   c. cystoscope
    b. urethrotome   d. cystometer

19. The medical term for the obstruction of the urethra is:
    a. urethropexy   c. urethrophraxis
    b. urethrospasm   d. urethrotome

20. All of the following terms refer to the process of emptying
    the bladder except:
    a. micturition   c. void
    b. urochrome   d. urination

21. The normal color of urine is:
    a. red   c. yellow to amber
    b. orange   d. greenish-yellow

22. Under chemical examination, the presence of _____ in the urine is an important sign of renal disease, acute glomerulonephritis and pyelonephritis.
    a. glucose
    b. protein
    c. bilirubin
    d. nitrites

23. The prefix olig means:
    a. against
    b. excessive
    c. water
    d. scanty

24. The word root stom means:
    a. new opening
    b. mouth
    c. stone
    d. pus

25. The suffix -dynia means:
    a. pain
    b. process
    c. paralysis
    d. disease

PART II MATCHING
DIRECTIONS: Using the answer sheet, write the letter of the definition that best matches the word.

26. anuria
27. cystogram
28. diuresis
29. enuresis
30. hematuria
31. incontinence
32. meatal
33. polyuria
34. uremia
35. ureterostenosis
36. renal failure
37. specific gravity
38. sterile
39. urea
40. urochrome

A. The presence of blood in the urine
B. The pigment that gives urine its normal color
C. Without the formation of urine
D. Excessive urination
E. A compound found in urine, blood, and lymph
F. A condition of increased flow of urine
G. A state of being free from living microorganisms
H. An x-ray record of the bladder
I. The inability to hold urine
J. The cessation of proper functioning of the kidney
K. Bedwetting
L. Pertaining to a passage
M. The weight of a substance compared with an equal amount of water
N. A condition of excessive urea in the blood
O. A condition of deficient urea in the blood
P. A condition of narrowing of the ureter

85

PART III FILL-IN-THE-BLANK
DIRECTIONS: Using the answer sheet, write the correct abbreviation for each of the following.

41. _____ antidiuretic hormone
42. _____ blood urea nitrogen
43. _____ chronic renal failure
44. _____ culture and sensitivity
45. _____ genitourinary
46. _____ water
47. _____ intake and output
48. _____ intravenous pyelogram
49. _____ kidney, ureter, and bladder
50. _____ phenylketonuria

THE URINARY SYSTEM
CHAPTER 10
POST TEST A

ANSWER KEY:

1.	c	26.	C
2.	d	27.	H
3.	a	28.	F
4.	b	29.	K
5.	c	30.	A
6.	b	31.	I
7.	d	32.	L
8.	a	33.	D
9.	d	34.	N
10.	b	35.	P
11.	d	36.	J
12.	a	37.	M
13.	b	38.	G
14.	a	39.	E
15.	d	40.	B
16.	b	41.	ADH
17.	c	42.	BUN
18.	a	43.	CRF
19.	c	44.	C&S
20.	b	45.	GU
21.	c	46.	H_2O
22.	b	47.	I&O
23.	d	48.	IVP
24.	b	49.	KUB
25.	a	50.	PKU

THE URINARY SYSTEM
CHAPTER 10
POST TEST B

PART I WORD PARTS
DIRECTIONS: Using the answer sheet, write the letter of the definition that best matches the word part.

1. hydro
2. olig
3. albumin
4. cysto
5. glycos
6. litho
7. meato
8. micturit
9. nephro
10. noct
11. pyelo
12. ureter
13. urethra
14. uro
15. -ectasia
16. -ectasy
17. -ist
18. -phraxis
19. -plegia
20. -ptosis
21. -rrhaphy
22. -scopy
23. -staxia
24. -tony
25. -trophy

A. sweet, sugar
B. to urinate
C. renal pelvis
D. urine
E. distention
F. kidney
G. one who specializes
H. paralysis
I. water
J. stone
K. prolapse, drooping
L. to view, examine
M. scanty
N. dripping, trickling
O. ureter
P. tension
Q. protein
R. nourishment, development
S. instrument
T. bladder
U. suture
V. to obstruct
W. passage
X. dilation
Y. urethra
Z. night

PART II FILL-IN-THE-BLANK
DIRECTIONS: Using the answer sheet, write the correct abbreviation or meaning for each of the following.

26. antidiuretic hormone
27. BUN
28. clean catch
29. cystometrogram
30. ESRD
31. HD
32. intravenous pyelogram
33. KUB
34. Na
35. UA

PART III MULTIPLE CHOICE

DIRECTIONS: Select the best answer to each multiple choice question and write the appropriate letter on the answer sheet.

36. The crushing of a kidney stone is called:
    a. lithotripsy
    b. lithotriptor
    c. lithotomy
    d. lithotome

37. The structural and functional unit of the kidney is the:
    a. nephron
    b. glomerulus
    c. neuron
    d. cortex

38. An average daily urinary output is approximately:
    a. 1200-1600 mL
    b. 1000-1500 mL
    c. 800-1200 mL
    d. 1400-1800 mL

39. A urine that has a fruity sweet odor may indicate:
    a. diabetes insipidus
    b. pyelonephritis
    c. dehydration
    d. diabetes mellitus

40. Urine has a specific gravity of:
    a. 1.000-1.020
    b. 1.002-1.020
    c. 1.015-1.025
    d. 1.020-1.040

41. A medication that decreases urine secretion is called:
    a. antidiuretic
    b. diuretic
    c. antibiotic
    d. antiemetic

42. _____ is excessive urination at night.
    a. Nocturia
    b. Oliguria
    c. Polyuria
    d. Pyuria

43. The external opening of the urethra is the:
    a. medulla
    b. meatus
    c. cortex
    d. trigone

44. The normal color of urine is:
    a. red
    b. orange
    c. yellow
    d. green

45. Difficult or painful urination is called:
    a. anuria
    b. dysuria
    c. enuresis
    d. nocturia

46. A urine test performed to determine the glomerular filtration rate is:
    a. BUN
    b. creatinine
    c. creatinine clearance
    d. KUB

47. A urine test performed to determine the presence of microorganisms is:
   a. BUN
   b. creatinine
   c. urine culture
   d. KUB

48. A test performed to visualize the kidneys, ureters, and bladder is:
   a. cystoscopy
   b. renal biopsy
   c. KUB
   d. intravenous pyelography

49. The use of high-frequency sound waves to visualize the kidneys is:
   a. retrograde pyelography
   b. intravenous pyelography
   c. ultrasonography
   d. cystoscopy

50. A flat-plate x-ray of the abdomen to indicate the size and position of the kidneys, ureters, and bladder is called:
   a. cystoscopy
   b. KUB
   c. BUN
   d. retrograde pyelography

THE URINARY SYSTEM
CHAPTER 10
POST TEST B

ANSWER KEY:

1.	I		26.	ADH
2.	M		27.	blood urea nitrogen
3.	Q		28.	CC
4.	T		29.	CMG
5.	A		30.	end-stage renal disease
6.	J		31.	hemodialysis
7.	W		32.	IVP
8.	B		33.	kidney, ureter, bladder
9.	F		34.	sodium
10.	Z		35.	urinalysis
11.	C		36.	a
12.	O		37.	a
13.	Y		38.	b
14.	D		39.	d
15.	E		40.	c
16.	X		41.	a
17.	G		42.	a
18.	V		43.	b
19.	H		44.	c
20.	K		45.	b
21.	U		46.	c
22.	L		47.	c
23.	N		48.	d
24.	P		49.	c
25.	R		50.	b

THE ENDOCRINE SYSTEM
CHAPTER 11
POST TEST A

PART I MULTIPLE CHOICE
DIRECTIONS: Select the best answer to each multiple choice question and write the appropriate letter on the answer sheet.

1. The _____ gland is known as the master gland of the body.
    a. pineal   c. pituitary
    b. thyroid   d. adrenal

2. Prolactin is secreted by the:
    a. neurohypophysis   c. ovaries
    b. pineal gland   d. adenohypophysis

3. The _____ gland plays a vital role in metabolism and regulates the body's metabolic processes.
    a. thyroid   c. pineal
    b. parathyroid   d. pituitary

4. _____ is essential for maintenance of a normal level of blood sugar.
    a. Cortisol   c. Parahormone
    b. Insulin   d. Serotonin

5. The principle mineralocorticoid secreted by the adrenal cortex is:
    a. aldosterone   c. oxytocin
    b. androgen   d. dopamine

6. All are true statements concerning epinephrine except:
    a. it elevates the systolic blood pressure
    b. it decreases the heart rate and cardiac output
    c. it dilates the bronchial tubes
    d. it dilates the pupils

7. An enlargement of the extremities due to excessive growth hormone is called:
    a. cretinism   c. acromegaly
    b. dwarfism   d. gigantism

8. The medical term for softening of a gland is:
    a. adenoma   c. adenosis
    b. adenomalacia   d. adenosclerosis

9. _____ is any disease of the adrenal gland.
    a. Adrenopathy   c. Adrenotropic
    b. Adenopathy   d. Adenalgia

10. A congenital deficiency in secretion of the thyroid hormone
    is called:
    a. diabetes   c. gigantism
    b. hirsutism   d. cretinism

11. A physician who specializes in the study of the endocrine
    system is known as a/an:
    a. endocrinology   c. pathologist
    b. endocrinologist   d. gastroenterologist

12. _____ means an abnormal protrusion of the eye.
    a. Exopthalmic   c. Exophthalmic
    b. Exocrine   d. Endocrine

13. Excessive secretion of milk after cessation of nursing is:
    a. galactorrhea   c. glandular
    b. mammorrhea   d. galactin

14. The medical term for pertaining to drowsiness, sluggish is:
    a. pallor   c. ascites
    b. myxedema   d. lethargic

15. The pituitary gland is also known as the:
    a. pineal   c. parathyroid
    b. hypophysis   d. pituitarism

16. _____ is a condition of premature old age occurring in
    children.
    a. Virilism   c. Progeria
    b. Progesterone   d. Vasopressin

17. A tumor of the islands of Langerhans is:
    a. insulitis   c. insulinoid
    b. insuloma   d. insulopathic

18. The surgical excision of the thyroid gland is called:
    a. thyroidotomy   c. thyrotherapy
    b. thyroidotome   d. thyroidectomy

19. _____ are biochemical substances, epinephrine,
    norepinephrine and dopamine.
    a. Catecholamines   c. Hormones
    b. Steroids   d. Iodines

20. The word root creat means:
    a. cretin   c. milk
    b. secrete   d. flesh

21. The word root kal means:
    a. calcium   c. potassium
    b. iron   d. magnesium

22. The suffix -ptosis means:
    a. fixation   c. disease
    b. drooping   d. resemble

23. The ovaries produce all of the following except:
    a. androgen   c. progesterone
    b. estrogen   d. estrone

24. _____ is a gland that produces an internal secretion.
    a. Exocrine   c. Ectropion
    b. Enzyme   d. Endocrine

25. _____ is used as an anti-inflammatory agent.
    a. Aldosterone   c. Dopamine
    b. Cortisone   d. Somatotropin

PART II MATCHING
DIRECTIONS: Using the answer sheet, write the letter of the definition that best matches the word.

26. adenoma
27. adrenal
28. diabetes
29. gigantism
30. hirsutism
31. hyperkalemia
32. hypogonadism
33. oxytocin
34. parathyroid
35. thyroid
36. virilism
37. vasopressin
38. epinephrine
39. dwarfism
40. testosterone

A. Also called ADH
B. A condition of being abnormally small
C. Stimulates uterine contraction during childbirth
D. A condition of being abnormally large
E. Excessive amounts of potassium in the blood
F. A tumor of a gland
G. Also called adrenaline
H. Toward the kidney
I. Male sex hormone
J. Masculinity developed in a female
K. Hairy condition
L. To go through
M. Deficient internal secretion of the gonads
N. Located beside the thyroid gland
O. Resembling a shield
P. Masculinity developed in a male

PART III FILL-IN-THE-BLANK

DIRECTIONS: Using the answer sheet, write the correct abbreviation for each of the following.

41. _____ adrenocorticotropic hormone
42. _____ basal metabolic rate
43. _____ diabetes mellitus
44. _____ follicle-stimulating hormone
45. _____ growth hormone
46. _____ somatotropin hormone
47. _____ triiodothyronine
48. _____ thyroxine
49. _____ thyroid function studies
50. _____ thyroid-stimulating hormone

THE ENDOCRINE SYSTEM
CHAPTER 11
POST TEST A

ANSWER KEY:

1.	c	26.	F
2.	d	27.	H
3.	a	28.	L
4.	b	29.	D
5.	a	30.	K
6.	b	31.	E
7.	c	32.	M
8.	b	33.	C
9.	a	34.	N
10.	d	35.	O
11.	b	36.	J
12.	c	37.	A
13.	a	38.	G
14.	d	39.	B
15.	b	40.	I
16.	c	41.	ACTH
17.	b	42.	BMR
18.	d	43.	DM
19.	a	44.	FSH
20.	d	45.	GH
21.	c	46.	STH
22.	b	47.	T_3
23.	a	48.	T_4
24.	d	49.	TFS
25.	b	50.	TSH

THE ENDOCRINE SYSTEM
CHAPTER 11
POST TEST B

PART I WORD PARTS

DIRECTIONS: Using the answer sheet, write the letter of the definition that best matches the word part.

1. ex
2. para
3. pro
4. acro
5. adeno
6. creat
7. crino
8. dwarf
9. galacto
10. gigant
11. hirsut
12. kal
13. letharg
14. myx
15. pituitar
16. thymo
17. thyro
18. viril
19. -betes
20. -oid
21. -osis
22. -physis
23. -ptosis
24. -therapy
25. -tome

A. gland
B. milk
C. potassium
D. beside
E. phlegm
F. to go
G. condition of
H. out, away from
I. extremity
J. giant
K. resemble
L. growth
M. before
N. drowsiness
O. thymus
P. drooping
Q. instrument to cut
R. flesh
S. treatment
T. excision
U. to secrete
V. thyroid, shield
W. masculine
X. small
Y. hairy
Z. mucus

PART II FILL-IN-THE-BLANK

DIRECTIONS: Using the answer sheet, write the correct abbreviation or meaning for each of the following.

26. ADH
27. diabetes mellitus
28. GTT
29. protein bound iodine
30. RIA

31. T_3
32. T_4
33. fasting blood sugar
34. vasopressin
35. BG

DIRECTIONS: Select the best answer to each multiple choice question and write the appropriate letter on the answer sheet.

36. _____ is known as the master gland.
    a. Pineal   c. Pituitary
    b. Thyroid   d. Adrenal

37. The _____ gland plays a vital role in metabolism.
    a. thyroid   c. pineal
    b. parathyroid   d. pituitary

38. An enlargement of the extremities due to excessive growth hormone is called:
    a. cretinism   c. acromegaly
    b. dwarfism   d. gigantism

39. A congenital deficiency in secretion of the thyroid hormone is called:
    a. diabetes   c. gigantism
    b. hirsutism   d. cretinism

40. _____ means an abnormal protrusion of the eye.
    a. Exopthalmic   c. Exophthalmic
    b. Exocrine   d. Endocrine

41. Excessive secretion of milk after cessation of nursing is:
    a. galactorrhea   c. glandular
    b. mammorrhea   d. galactin

42. The medical term for drowsiness is:
    a. pallor   c. ascites
    b. myxedema   d. lethargic

43. The pituitary gland is also known as the:
    a. pineal   c. parathyroid
    b. hypophysis   d. pituitarism

44. _____ is a condition of premature old age occurring in children.
    a. Virilism   c. Progeria
    b. Progesterone   d. Vasopressin

45. A tumor of the islands of Langerhans is called:
    a. insulitis   c. insulinoid
    b. insuloma   d. insulopathic

46. A test performed on urine to determine the amount of epinephrine and norepinephrine present is:
    a. catecholamines   c. protein bound iodine
    b. corticotropin   d. total calcium

47. Increased levels may indicate diabetes mellitus:
   a. thyroid scan   c. fasting blood sugar
   b. total calcium   d. protein bound iodine

48. A test used to detect tumors of the thyroid gland is:
   a. thyroxine   c. thyroid scan
   b. total calcium   d. protein bound iodine

49. A blood sugar test that is performed at specified intervals
    after the patient has taken glucose is:
   a. fasting blood sugar
   b. glucose tolerance test
   c. protein bound iodine
   d. corticotropin

50. A test used in the diagnosing of adrenal tumors is called:
   a. 17-HCS   c. 17-KS
   b. 17-OHCS   d. 17-HDL

THE ENDOCRINE SYSTEM
CHAPTER 11
POST TEST B

ANSWER KEY:

1.	H	26.	antidiuretic hormone
2.	D	27.	DM
3.	M	28.	glucose tolerance test
4.	I	29.	PBI
5.	A	30.	radioimmunoassay
6.	R	31.	triiodothyronine
7.	U	32.	thyroxine
8.	X	33.	FBS
9.	B	34.	VP
10.	J	35.	blood glucose
11.	Y	36.	c
12.	C	37.	a
13.	N	38.	c
14.	Z	39.	d
15.	E	40.	c
16.	O	41.	a
17.	V	42.	d
18.	W	43.	b
19.	F	44.	c
20.	K	45.	b
21.	G	46.	a
22.	L	47.	c
23.	P	48.	c
24.	S	49.	b
25.	Q	50.	c

THE NERVOUS SYSTEM
CHAPTER 12
POST TEST A

PART I MULTIPLE CHOICE
DIRECTIONS: Select the best answer to each multiple choice
question and write the appropriate letter on the answer sheet.

1. The brain and spinal cord constitute the _____ nervous
    system.
    a. peripheral   c. autonomic
    b. central   d. sympathetic

2. _____ function to mediate impulses between sensory and
    motor neurons.
    a. Axons   c. Interneurons
    b. Dendrites   d. Neurons

3. Nerves that transmit impulses to the CNS are called:
    a. sensory   c. peripheral
    b. motor   d. autonomic

4. Which of the following is not a membrane that encloses the
    brain?
    a. dura mater   c. pia mater
    b. arachnoid   d. oblongata

5. The brain's major motor area is located in the:
    a. parietal lobe   c. temporal lobe
    b. frontal lobe   d. occipital lobe

6. Which lobe contains centers for auditory and language input?
    a. parietal   c. temporal
    b. frontal   d. occipital

7. Which of the following is not a function of the hypothalamus?
    a. it acts as a regulator
    b. it coordinates movement
    c. it produces neurosecretions
    d. it produces hormones

8. The medulla oblongata regulates and controls all of the
    following except:
    a. breathing   c. vomiting
    b. swallowing   d. temperature

9. An abnormal fear of high places is called:
    a. acrophobia   c. aerophobia
    b. agoraphobia   d. autophobia

10. A condition where there is a loss of memory is called:
    a. amentia   c. amnesia
    b. analgesia   d. anesthesia

11. The medical term for the loss of the ability to eat is:
    a. aphasia   c. asthenia
    b. apraxia   d. aphagia

12. A condition of imperfect development of the spinal cord is:
    a. atelomyelia   c. ataxia
    b. atelencephalia   d. anencephaly

13. The medical term for a headache is:
    a. chorea   c. cerebromalacia
    b. coryza   d. cephalalgia

14. The surgical incision into the skull is:
    a. craniectomy   c. craniocele
    b. craniotomy   d. cranioplasty

15. Difficulty in comprehending the written language is called:
    a. dysphasia   c. diplegia
    b. dysthymia   d. dyslexia

16. Paralysis that affects one side of the body is called:
    a. apraxia   c. hemiparesis
    b. paraplegia   d. quadriplegia

17. An artificially induced sleep is known as:
    a. hypnosis   c. stupor
    b. coma   d. hypnology

18. A thin membranous sheath that envelops a nerve fiber is:
    a. neuron   c. neurilemma
    b. neuroblast   d. neurocyte

19. The surgical crushing of a nerve is called:
    a. neurotripsy   c. neuroma
    b. neurotomy   d. neurolysis

20. The medical term for swelling of the optic disk is:
    a. phagomania   c. paranoia
    b. papilledema   d. paresthesia

21. _____ is a chromaffin cell tumor of the adrenal medulla.
    a. Astrocytoma   c. Pheochromocytoma
    b. Glioma   d. Neuroblastoma

22. _____ is a division of spinal nerve roots.
    a. Radiculitis   c. Rachiomyelitis
    b. Radicotomy   d. Cordotomy

23. The medical term that means an interrelationship of the mind and the body is:
   a. somatic
   b. psychosis
   c. somnambulism
   d. psychosomatic

24. A severe form of senile dementia that may be due to a defect in the neurotransmitter system is called:
   a. anorexia nervosa
   b. myasthenia gravis
   c. Alzheimer's disease
   d. multiple sclerosis

25. A cerebrovascular accident may be called all of the following except:
   a. autism
   b. stroke
   c. CVA
   d. apoplexy

PART II MATCHING
DIRECTIONS: Using the answer sheet, write the letter of the definition that best matches the word.

26. analgesia
27. asthenia
28. ataxia
29. bradykinesia
30. coma
31. cerebromalacia
32. craniectomy
33. diskectomy
34. endorphin
35. egocentric
36. glioma
37. hydrocephalus
38. laminectomy
39. bulimia
40. syncope

A. Binge eating
B. Being self-centered
C. Fainting
D. Lack of the sense of pain
E. Abnormal slowness of motion
F. Excision of an intervertebral disk
G. Excision of a vertebral posterior arch
H. Loss of strength
I. An increased amount of fluid within the brain
J. Loss of muscular coordination
K. A tumor composed of neuroglial tissue
L. An unconscious state
M. Natural analgesic
N. Softening of the cerebrum
O. Hardening of the cerebrum
P. Excision of a portion of the skull

PART III FILL-IN-THE-BLANK
DIRECTIONS: Using the answer sheet, write the correct
abbreviation for each of the following.

41. _____ amyotrophic lateral sclerosis
42. _____ chronic brain syndrome
43. _____ cerebral palsy
44. _____ cerebrovascular accident
45. _____ electroencephalogram
46. _____ herniated disk syndrome
47. _____ intracranial pressure
48. _____ mental retardation
49. _____ nerve conduction velocity
50. _____ pneumoencephalography

THE NERVOUS SYSTEM
CHAPTER 12
POST TEST A

ANSWER KEY:

1.	b	26.	D
2.	c	27.	H
3.	a	28.	J
4.	d	29.	E
5.	b	30.	L
6.	c	31.	N
7.	b	32.	P
8.	d	33.	F
9.	a	34.	M
10.	c	35.	B
11.	d	36.	K
12.	a	37.	I
13.	d	38.	G
14.	b	39.	A
15.	d	40.	C
16.	c	41.	ALS
17.	a	42.	CBS
18.	c	43.	CP
19.	a	44.	CVA
20.	b	45.	EEG
21.	c	46.	HDS
22.	b	47.	ICP
23.	d	48.	MR
24.	c	49.	NCV
25.	a	50.	PEG

THE NERVOUS SYSTEM
CHAPTER 12
POST TEST B

PART I WORD PARTS
DIRECTIONS: Using the answer sheet, write the letter of the definition that best matches the word part.

1.	astro	A.	cerebrum
2.	hemi	B.	I, self
3.	infra	C.	lobe
4.	supra	D.	nerve
5.	atelo	E.	mind
6.	cerebro	F.	feeling
7.	chromo	G.	star-shaped
8.	ego	H.	brain
9.	encephalo	I.	word
10.	hypno	J.	root
11.	lobo	K.	a sheath, husk
12.	logo	L.	half
13.	meningo	M.	color
14.	myelo	N.	madness
15.	neuro	O.	softening
16.	pheo	P.	below
17.	psycho	Q.	memory
18.	rachio	R.	above
19.	radicul	S.	spine
20.	spondylo	T.	strength
21.	-esthesia	U.	sleep
22.	-mania	V.	membrane
23.	-mnesia	W.	dusky
24.	-lemma	X.	vertebra
25.	-sthenia	Y.	spinal cord
		Z.	imperfect

PART II FILL-IN-THE-BLANK
DIRECTIONS: Using the answer sheet, write the correct abbreviation or meaning for each of the following.

26. AD
27. computerized tomography
28. CVA
29. electric shock therapy
30. HDS

31. lumbar puncture
32. multiple sclerosis
33. PEG
34. PET
35. TENS

PART III MULTIPLE CHOICE

DIRECTIONS: Select the best answer to each multiple choice question and write the appropriate letter on the answer sheet.

36. Amyotrophic lateral sclerosis is also known as:
    a. apoplexy   c. autism
    b. Lou Gehrig's disease   d. Alzheimer's disease

37. _____ are chemical substances that act as natural analgesics.
    a. Acetylcholines   c. Endorphins
    b. Biogenic amines   d. Receptors

38. The medical term for fainting is:
    a. sciatica   c. narcolepsy
    b. syncope   d. palsy

39. The _____ nervous system consists of the brain and spinal cord.
    a. peripheral   c. autonomic
    b. central   d. sympathetic

40. All of the following membranes enclose the brain except:
    a. dura mater   c. pia mater
    b. arachnoid   d. oblongata

41. Which lobe is the brain's major motor area?
    a. parietal   c. temporal
    b. frontal   d. occipital

42. Difficulty in comprehending the written language is called:
    a. dysphasia   c. diplegia
    b. dysthymia   d. dyslexia

43. _____ is the surgical incision into the skull.
    a. Craniectomy   c. Craniocele
    b. Craniotomy   d. Cranioplasty

44. The medical term for headache is:
    a. chorea   c. cerebromalacia
    b. coryza   d. cephalalgia

45. The medical term for the loss of the ability to eat is:
    a. aphasia   c. asthenia
    b. apraxia   d. aphagia

46. A diagnostic procedure used to study the structure of the brain is called:
    a. computed tomography   c. electroencephalography
    b. echoencephalography   d. myelogram

47. The process of using ultrasound to determine the presence of a centrally located mass in the brain is called:
   a. computed tomography   c. electroencephalography
   b. echoencephalography   d. myelogram

48. The x-ray of the spinal canal after the injection of a radiopaque dye is called:
   a. cerebral angiography
   b. computed tomography
   c. myelogram
   d. ultrasonography

49. A computer-based nuclear imaging procedure that can produce three-dimensional pictures of actual organ functioning is:
   a. electroencephalography
   b. myelogram
   c. ultrasonography
   d. positron emission tomography

50. The use of high-frequency sound waves to record echoes on an oscilloscope and film is:
   a. electroencephalography
   b. myelogram
   c. ultrasonography
   d. positron emission tomography

ANSWER KEY:

1.	G	26.	Alzheimer's disease
2.	L	27.	CT
3.	P	28.	cerebrovascular accident
4.	R	29.	EST
5.	Z	30.	herniated disk syndrome
6.	A	31.	LP
7.	M	32.	MS
8.	B	33.	pneumoencephalography
9.	H	34.	positron emission tomography
10.	U	35.	transcutaneous electrical
11.	C		nerve stimulation
12.	I	36.	b
13.	V	37.	c
14.	Y	38.	b
15.	D	39.	b
16.	W	40.	d
17.	E	41.	b
18.	S	42.	d
19.	J	43.	b
20.	X	44.	d
21.	F	45.	d
22.	N	46.	a
23.	Q	47.	b
24.	K	48.	c
25.	T	49.	d
		50.	c

**THE EAR
CHAPTER 13
POST TEST A**

PART I MULTIPLE CHOICE
DIRECTIONS: Select the best answer to each multiple choice
question and write the appropriate letter on the answer sheet.

1. The external ear consists of all of the following except:
    a. cochlea   c. auricle
    b. tympanic membrane   d. external acoustic meatus

2. Which structure of the external ear collects sound waves?
    a. cochlea   c. auricle
    b. tympanic membrane   d. external acoustic meatus

3. All of the following are ossicles of the middle ear except:
    a. malleus   c. utricle
    b. incus   d. stapes

4. The _____ is a bony structure located between the
    cochlea and the three semicircular canals.
    a. auricle   c. utricle
    b. vestibule   d. saccule

5. The auditory nerve is also known as the:
    a. 5th cranial nerve   c. 9th cranial nerve
    b. 7th cranial nerve   d. 8th cranial nerve

6. Located on the basilar membrane is the _____ containing
    hair cell sensory receptors for the sense of hearing.
    a. semicircular canals   c. organ of Corti
    b. cochlear duct   d. tympanic membrane

7. One who specializes in disorders of hearing is called a/an:
    a. audiologist   c. otolaryngologist
    b. laryngologist   d. otorhinolaryngologist

8. _____ is an instrument used to measure hearing.
    a. Otoscope   c. Audiometer
    b. Audiphone   d. Myringoscope

9. The clear fluid contained within the labyrinth of the ear is:
    a. perilymph   c. plasma
    b. cerumen   d. endolymph

10. Surgical excision of the tympanic membrane is called:
    a. myringotomy   c. myringectomy
    b. myringoplasty   d. myringotome

11. The medical term for earache is:
    a. mastoidalgia   c. otic
    b. otodynia   d. otitis

12. _____ is a fungus condition of the ear.
    a. Otomycosis   c. Otosclerosis
    b. Otopyorrhea   d. Otolith

13. Serum fluid of the inner ear is called:
    a. endolymph   c. plasma
    b. cerumen   d. perilymph

14. A ringing sound in the ear is called:
    a. vertigo   c. presbycusis
    b. tinnitus   d. tympanitis

15. _____ is a state of balance.
    a. Epilation   c. Equatorial
    b. Equivalence   d. Equilibrium

16. The _____ is located between the middle ear and the
    throat and serves to equalize pressure on both sides of the
    eardrum.
    a. eustachian tube   c. auditory canal
    b. tympanic membrane   d. oval window

17. The prefix peri means:
    a. across   c. within
    b. through   d. around

18. The word root presby means:
    a. hard   c. old
    b. soft   d. fat

19. The suffix -cusis means:
    a. voice   c. sound
    b. hearing   d. noise

20. All of the following terms are spelled correctly except:
    a. acoustic   c. labryinthitis
    b. tympanic   d. otosclerosis

21. The medical term _____ means pertaining to the sense of
    hearing.
    a. aural   c. endaural
    b. auditory   d. audiology

22. An instrument used for cutting the eardrum is:
    a. myringoscope   c. myringotomy
    b. myringoplasty   d. myringotome

23. Impairment of hearing occurring in old age is called:
    a. tinnitus   c. vertigo
    b. presbycusis   d. tympanitis

24. The medical term for earwax is:
    a. cerumen   c. perilymph
    b. cochlea   d. endolymph

25. Complete or partial loss of the ability to hear is:
    a. blindness   c. vitiligo
    b. mute   d. deafness

PART II MATCHING
DIRECTIONS: Using the answer sheet, write the letter of the
definition that best matches the word.

26. myringoplasty   A. The middle of the three
27. otitis   ossicles; the anvil
28. otolaryngologist   B. Pertaining to both ears
29. labyrinth   C. Dizziness, lightheadedness
30. otopyorrhea   D. The eardrum
31. otorhinolaryngology   E. Inflammation of the ear
32. monaural   F. The inner ear
33. tympanic   G. A small, saclike structure
34. auricle   H. One who specializes in the
35. binaural   study of the ear and larynx
36. cochlea   I. External portion of the ear
37. fenestration   J. Surgical repair of the tympanic
38. incus   membrane
39. utricle   K. Pertaining to one ear
40. vertigo   L. The process of making a new
                               opening in the labyrinth
                           M. Flow of pus from the ear
                           N. Contains the organ of hearing
                           O. The study of the ear, nose, and
                               larynx
                           P. The study of the ear, nose, and
                               pharynx

PART III FILL-IN-THE-BLANK
DIRECTIONS: Using the answer sheet, write the correct
abbreviation for each of the following
41. _____ air conduction
42. _____ right ear
43. _____ left ear
44. _____ both ears
45. _____ decibel
46. _____ eyes, ears, nose, throat
47. _____ otitis media
48. _____ serous otitis media
49. _____ bone conduction
50. _____ usual childhood diseases

ANSWER KEY:

1.	a	26.	J
2.	c	27.	E
3.	c	28.	H
4.	b	29.	F
5.	d	30.	M
6.	c	31.	O
7.	a	32.	K
8.	c	33.	D
9.	d	34.	I
10.	c	35.	B
11.	b	36.	N
12.	a	37.	L
13.	d	38.	A
14.	b	39.	G
15.	d	40.	C
16.	a	41.	AC
17.	d	42.	AD
18.	c	43.	AS
19.	b	44.	AU
20.	c	45.	db
21.	b	46.	EENT
22.	d	47.	OM
23.	b	48.	SOM
24.	a	49.	BC
25.	d	50.	UCHD

PART I WORD PARTS
DIRECTIONS: Using the answer sheet, write the letter of the definition that best matches the word part.

1.	endo	A.	ear
2.	peri	B.	hardening
3.	audio	C.	maze
4.	cochleo	D.	drum
5.	labyrintho	E.	hearing
6.	laryngo	F.	voice
7.	myringo	G.	measurement
8.	oto	H.	old
9.	pharynge	I.	within
10.	phone	J.	pus
11.	presby	K.	flow
12.	pyo	L.	resemble
13.	rhino	M.	around
14.	scler	N.	fat
15.	staped	O.	incision
16.	steat	P.	a jingling
17.	tinnit	Q.	to hear
18.	tympan	R.	larynx
19.	-cusis	S.	stone
20.	-lith	T.	pharynx
21.	-lymph	U.	nose
22.	-metry	V.	pertaining to
23.	-rrhea	W.	land snail
24.	-tomy	X.	serum, clear fluid
25.	-us	Y.	stirrup
		Z.	drum membrane

PART II FILL-IN-THE-BLANK
DIRECTIONS: Using the answer sheet, write the correct abbreviation or meaning for each of the following.

26.	right ear	31.	OM
27.	left ear	32.	serous otitis media
28.	both ears	33.	usual childhood diseases
29.	EENT	34.	AC
30.	HD	35.	BC

PART III MULTIPLE CHOICE
DIRECTIONS: Select the best answer to each multiple choice question and write the appropriate letter on the answer sheet.

36. The medical term for earwax is:
    a. cerumen   c. perilymph
    b. cochlea   d. endolymph

37. Complete or partial loss of the ability to hear is:
    a. blindness   c. vitiligo
    b. muteness   d. deafness

38. _____ is a fungus condition of the ear.
    a. Otomycosis   c. Otosclerosis
    b. Otopyorrhea   d. Otolith

39. Serum fluid of the inner ear is called:
    a. endolymph   c. plasma
    b. cerumen   d. perilymph

40. A ringing sound in the ear is called:
    a. vertigo   c. presbycusis
    b. tinnitus   d. tympanitis

41. _____ is a state of balance.
    a. Epilation   c. Equatorial
    b. Equivalence   d. Equilibrium

42. An instrument used to measure hearing is called:
    a. otoscope   c. audiometer
    b. audiphone   d. myringoscope

43. The clear fluid contained within the labyrinth is called:
    a. perilymph   c. plasma
    b. cerumen   d. endolymph

44. Surgical excision of the tympanic membrane is:
    a. myringotomy   c. myringectomy
    b. myringoplasty   d. myringotome

45. The medical term for earache is:
    a. mastoidalgia   c. otic
    b. otodynia   d. otitis

46. The response to auditory stimuli that can be measured independent of the patients's subjective response is:
    a. auditory evoked response
    b. electronystagmography
    c. falling test
    d. otoscopy

115

47. A recording of eye movement in response to specific stimuli
    is known as:
    a. auditory evoked response
    b. electronystagmography
    c. falling test
    d. otoscopy

48. A test used to observe the patient for marked swaying is:
    a. auditory evoked response
    b. electronystagmography
    c. falling test
    d. otoscopy

49. The visual examination of the external auditory canal and the
    tympanic membrane is:
    a. tuning fork test   c. electronystagmography
    b. tympanometry   d. otoscopy

50. The measurement of the movement of the tympanic membrane is:
    a. tuning fork test   c. otoscopy
    b. tympanometry   d. past-pointing test

ANSWER KEY:

1.	I	26.	AD
2.	M	27.	AS
3.	Q	28.	AU
4.	W	29.	eyes, ears, nose, throat
5.	C	30.	hearing distance
6.	R	31.	otitis media
7.	Z	32.	SOM
8.	A	33.	UCHD
9.	T	34.	air conduction
10.	F	35.	bone conduction
11.	H	36.	a
12.	J	37.	d
13.	U	38.	a
14.	B	39.	d
15.	Y	40.	b
16.	N	41.	d
17.	P	42.	c
18.	D	43.	d
19.	E	44.	c
20.	S	45.	b
21.	X	46.	a
22.	G	47.	b
23.	K	48.	c
24.	O	49.	d
25.	V	50.	b

THE EYE
CHAPTER 14
POST TEST A

PART I MULTIPLE CHOICE
DIRECTIONS: Select the best answer to each multiple choice
question and write the appropriate letter on the answer sheet.

1. The _____ is the anterior transparent portion of the
    eyeball.
    a. sclera   c. retina
    b. cornea   d. iris

2. All of the following make up the external structure of the
    eye except:
    a. uvea   c. eyelids
    b. orbit   d. conjunctiva

3. The process of sharpening the focus of light on the retina is
    known as:
    a. vision   c. accommodation
    b. contraction   d. dilation

4. The _____ is the opening in the center of the iris.
    a. pupil   c. sclera
    b. retina   d. cornea

5. The colored membrane attached to the ciliary body is:
    a. cornea   c. iris
    b. pupil   d. sclera

6. An involuntary, constant, rhythmic movement of the eyeball
    is called:
    a. strabismus   c. pterygium
    b. trichiasis   d. nystagmus

7. The medical term for dullness of vision is:
    a. amblyopia   c. ametropia
    b. diplopia   d. aphakia

8. Drooping of the upper eyelids is called:
    a. blepharitis   c. chalazion
    b. blepharoptosis   d. conjunctivitis

9. The process of turning outward, as the edges of the eyelid
    is known as:
    a. emmetropia   c. esotropia
    b. ectropion   d. anisocoria

10. An instrument used to measure intraocular pressure is:
    a. gonioscope   c. optomyometer
    b. keratometer   d. tonometer

11. The medical term for night blindness is:
    a. myopia   c. nyctalopia
    b. retinoblastoma   d. amblyopia

12. A malignant tumor of the germ cell of the retina is:
    a. retinitis   c. retinopathy
    b. retinoblastoma   d. retinal

13. An opacity of the crystalline lens is called:
    a. chalazion   c. trichiasis
    b. glaucoma   d. cataract

14. The medical term for farsightedness is:
    a. hyperopia   c. myopia
    b. diplopia   d. astigmatism

15. Surgical binding of part of the iris to form an artificial
    one is called:
    a. iridodesis   c. iridectomy
    b. iridocyclitis   d. iridotasis

16. A physician who specializes in the study of the eye is:
    a. ophthalmology   c. optician
    b. optometrist   d. ophthalmologist

17. A condition of hardening of the crystalline lens is called:
    a. phacolysis   c. presbyopia
    b. phacosclerosis   d. orthoptics

18. An unusual intolerance of light is known as:
    a. photophobia   c. strabismus
    b. photocoagulation   d. conjunctivitis

19. The suffix -itis means:
    a. condition of   c. disease
    b. inflammation   d. tumor

20. The prefix tri means:
    a. one   c. three
    b. two   d. four

21. The combining form kerato means:
    a. pupil   c. lens
    b. cornea   d. iris

22. Dryness of the conjunctiva is called:
    a. xenophthalmia   c. xerophthalmia
    b. chalazion   d. sty(e)

23. An agent that causes the pupil to dilate is called:
    a. miotic   c. hematinic
    b. oxytocic   d. mydriatic

24. The middle or vascular coat of the eye is called:
   a. iris   c. retina
   b. cornea   d. uvea

25. The medical term for normal vision is:
   a. hyperopia   c. myopia
   b. emmetropia   d. presbyopia

PART II MATCHING
DIRECTIONS: Using the answer sheet, write the letter of the definition that best matches the word.

26. blepharitis
27. choroiditis
28. cycloplegia
29. dacryocystitis
30. esotropia
31. keratitis
32. lacrimal
33. myopia
34. anomaloscope
35. glaucoma
36. chalazion
37. miotic
38. epiphora
39. strabismus
40. radial keratotomy

A. A small, hard cyst of a Meibomian gland
B. Inflammation of the cornea
C. A surgical procedure that may be performed to correct myopia
D. Inflammation of the edges of the eyelids
E. Instrument used for detecting color blindness
F. Crossed eyes
G. An agent that causes the pupil to contract
H. Inflammation of the vascular coat of the eye
I. The abnormal downpour of tears
J. Pertaining to tears
K. A squint
L. Paralysis of the ciliary muscles
M. Nearsightedness
N. Increased intraocular pressure
O. Inflammation of the tear sac
P. Decreased intraocular pressure

PART III FILL-IN-THE-BLANK
DIRECTIONS: Using the answer sheet, write the correct abbreviation for each of the following.

41. _____ distance visual acuity
42. _____ extraocular movement
43. _____ light and accommodation
44. _____ myopia
45. _____ near visual acuity
46. _____ right eye
47. _____ left eye
48. _____ both eyes
49. _____ pupils equal, react to light and accommodation
50. _____ rapid eye movement

ANSWER KEY:

1.	b	26.	D
2.	a	27.	H
3.	c	28.	L
4.	a	29.	O
5.	c	30.	F
6.	d	31.	B
7.	a	32.	J
8.	b	33.	M
9.	b	34.	E
10.	d	35.	N
11.	c	36.	A
12.	b	37.	G
13.	d	38.	I
14.	a	39.	K
15.	a	40.	C
16.	d	41.	DVA
17.	b	42.	EOM
18.	a	43.	L & A
19.	b	44.	MY
20.	c	45.	NVA
21.	b	46.	OD
22.	c	47.	OS
23.	d	48.	OU
24.	d	49.	PERLA
25.	b	50.	REM

THE EYE
CHAPTER 14
POST TEST B

PART I WORD PARTS
DIRECTION: Using the answer sheet, write the letter of the definition that best matches the word part.

1.	dipl	A.	dull
2.	bi	B.	iris
3.	em	C.	eye
4.	ec	D.	eyelid
5.	eso	E.	light
6.	ambly	F.	dry
7.	blepharo	G.	pertaining to
8.	cyclo	H.	destruction
9.	dacryo	I.	double
10.	irido	J.	ciliary body
11.	kerato	K.	stretching
12.	nyctal	L.	tone
13.	ophthalmo	M.	uvea
14.	phaco	N.	two
15.	photo	O.	retina
16.	retino	P.	pupil
17.	tono	Q.	in
18.	uve	R.	tear
19.	xen	S.	cornea
20.	xer	T.	binding
21.	-ary	U.	out
22.	-desis	V.	foreign material
23.	-graphy	W.	recording
24.	-lysis	X.	inward
25.	-tasis	Y.	blind
		Z.	lens

PART II FILL-IN-THE-BLANK
DIRECTIONS: Using the answer sheet, write the correct abbreviation or meaning for each of the following.

26. DVA
27. emmetropia
28. hypermetropia
    (hyperopia)
29. IOL
30. MY

31. right eye
32. left eye
33. both eyes

34. REM
35. ST

PART III MULTIPLE CHOICE
DIRECTIONS: Select the best answer to each multiple choice question and write the appropriate letter on the answer sheet.

36. The process of using ultrasound to disintegrate a cataract is known as:
    a. epiphora
    b. phacoemulsification
    c. trabeculoplasty
    d. enucleation

37. A surgical procedure that may be performed to correct myopia is known as:
    a. radial keratotomy
    b. photocoagulation
    c. phacoemulsification
    d. trabeculoplasty

38. An opacity of the crystalline lens is called:
    a. chalazion
    b. glaucoma
    c. trichiasis
    d. cataract

39. An instrument used to measure intraocular pressure is:
    a. gonioscope
    b. keratometer
    c. optomyometer
    d. tonometer

40. The medical term for dullness of vision is:
    a. amblyopia
    b. diplopia
    c. ametropia
    d. aphakia

41. An involuntary, constant, rhythmic movement of the eyeball is called:
    a. strabismus
    b. trichiasis
    c. pterygium
    d. nystagmus

42. The colored membrane attached to the ciliary body is:
    a. cornea
    b. pupil
    c. iris
    d. sclera

43. The opening in the center of the iris is:
    a. pupil
    b. retina
    c. sclera
    d. cornea

44. The process of sharpening the focus of light on the retina is known as:
    a. vision
    b. contraction
    c. accommodation
    d. dilation

45. The anterior transparent portion of the eyeball is:
    a. sclera
    b. cornea
    c. retina
    d. iris

46. The measurement of the forward protrusion of the eye is:
    a. gonioscopy
    b. keratometry
    c. exophthalmometry
    d. tonometry

47. The measurement of the cornea is called:
    a. gonioscopy   c. exophthalmometry
    b. keratometry   d. tonometry

48. _____ is used to identify changes in the blood vessels
    in the eye and to diagnose systemic diseases.
    a. Exophthalmometry   c. Ophthalmoscopy
    b. Gonioscopy   d. Tonometry

49. The measurement of the intraocular pressure of the eye is:
    a. exophthalmometry   c. ophthalmoscopy
    b. gonioscopy   d. tonometry

50. The measurement of the acuteness or sharpness of vision is:
    a. color vision test   c. tonometry
    b. ultrasonography   d. visual acuity

THE EYE
CHAPTER 14
POST TEST B

ANSWER KEY:

1.	I	26.	distance visual acuity
2.	N	27.	EM
3.	Q	28.	HT
4.	U	29.	intraocular lens
5.	X	30.	myopia
6.	A	31.	OD
7.	D	32.	OS
8.	J	33.	OU
9.	R	34.	rapid eye movement
10.	B	35.	esotropia
11.	S	36.	b
12.	Y	37.	a
13.	C	38.	d
14.	Z	39.	d
15.	E	40.	a
16.	O	41.	d
17.	L	42.	c
18.	M	43.	c
19.	V	44.	a
20.	F	45.	b
21.	G	46.	c
22.	T	47.	b
23.	W	48.	c
24.	H	49.	d
25.	K	50.	d

THE FEMALE REPRODUCTIVE SYSTEM
CHAPTER 15
POST TEST A

PART I MULTIPLE CHOICE
DIRECTIONS: Select the best answer to each multiple choice
question and write the appropriate letter on the answer sheet.

1. The following are identifiable areas of the uterus except:
   a. body   c. cortex
   b. isthmus   d. cervix

2. The finger-like processes that work to propel the discharged
   ovum into the tube are called:
   a. flagella   c. filum
   b. fimbriae   d. fillet

3. The process of bending forward of the uterus at its body and
   neck is called:
   a. anteflexion   c. anteversion
   b. retroflexion   d. retroversion

4. The external region between the vulva and the anus is:
   a. perineum   c. perineurium
   b. peritoneum   d. perinephrium

5. The medical term for a difficult monthly flow is:
   a. amenorrhea   c. dystocia
   b. dyspareunia   d. dysmenorrhea

6. _____ is the study of the female.
   a. Gynecologist   c. Genitalia
   b. Gynecology   d. Genioplasty

7. The process of obtaining pictures of the breast by the use of
   roentgen rays is called:
   a. mammoplasty   c. mammography
   b. mastitis   d. mastectomy

8. The cessation of the monthly flow is called:
   a. menorrhea   c. menorrhagia
   b. menopause   d. oligomenorrhea

9. The term for a woman who is bearing her first child is:
   a. primipara   c. nullipara
   b. multipara   d. unipara

10. The male or female reproductive organs are called:
    a. genial   c. genal
    b. genetics   d. genitalia

11. Surgical excision of the uterus is called:
    a. hysterotomy   c. hymenectomy
    b. hysterectomy   d. hysterorrhexis

12. A surgical procedure to prevent tearing of the perineum and
    to facilitate delivery of the fetus is called:
    a. eutocia   c. episiotomy
    b. colpotomy   d. hysterotomy

13. Inflammation of an ovary is known as:
    a. oogenesis   c. oophorectomy
    b. oophoritis   d. oophorotomy

14. The surgical excision of a fallopian tube is called:
    a. salpingectomy   c. salpingitis
    b. salpingostomy   d. salpingopexy

15. The term that means resulting from sexual intercourse is:
    a. menarche   c. secundines
    b. parturition   d. venereal

16. The developing young in the uterus from the third month to
    birth is called:
    a. embryo   c. zygote
    b. fetus   d. neonatal

17. The process in which an ovum is discharged from the cortex of
    the ovary is known as:
    a. mittelschmerz   c. quickening
    b. ovulation   d. menarche

18. The prefix pseudo means:
    a. false   c. none
    b. first   d. all

19. The prefix nulli means:
    a. none   c. new
    b. scanty   d. one

20. The word root partum means:
    a. month   c. turning
    b. receive   d. labor

21. The suffix -cyesis means:
    a. solution   c. pregnancy
    b. injection   d. flow

22. The suffix -metry means:
    a. measurement   c. recording
    b. instrument   d. process

23. Inflammation of the muscular wall of the uterus is:
    a. pyometritis   c. vaginitis
    b. myometritis   d. cervicitis

24. The _____ is a musculomembranous tube extending from the vestibule to the uterus.
    a. ovary   c. fallopian tube
    b. eustachian tube   d. vagina

25. The following terms are spelled correctly except:
    a. mensturation   c. parturition
    b. colostrum   d. amniocentesis

PART II MATCHING
DIRECTIONS: Using the answer sheet, write the letter of the definition that best matches the word.

26. abortion
27. ante partum
28. colporrhaphy
29. cystocele
30. dyspareunia
31. oligomenorrhea
32. zygote
33. pyosalpinx
34. trimester
35. vaginitis
36. secundines
37. lumpectomy
38. parturition
39. menarche
40. puerperium

A. Inflammation of the vagina
B. The afterbirth
C. 4-6 week period after childbirth
D. Surgical removal of a tumor from the breast
E. To miscarry
F. Hernia of the bladder that protrudes into the vagina
G. Beginning of the monthly flow
H. Time before the onset of labor
I. The act of giving birth
J. Suture of the vagina
K. A period of 3 months
L. The fertilized ovum
M. Painful sexual intercourse
N. Accumulation of pus in the fallopian tube
O. Scanty monthly flow
P. Heavy monthly flow

PART III FILL-IN-THE-BLANK
DIRECTIONS: Using the answer sheet, write the correct abbreviation for each of the following.
41. _____ abdominal hysterectomy
42. _____ cesarean section
43. _____ dilation (dilatation) and curettage
44. _____ expected date of confinement
45. _____ follicle-stimulating hormone
46. _____ gynecology
47. _____ obstetrics
48. _____ last menstrual period
49. _____ Papanicolaou (smear)
50. _____ pelvic inflammatory disease

THE FEMALE REPRODUCTIVE SYSTEM
CHAPTER 15
POST TEST A

ANSWER KEY:

1.	c	26.	E
2.	b	27.	H
3.	a	28.	J
4.	a	29.	F
5.	d	30.	M
6.	b	31.	O
7.	c	32.	L
8.	b	33.	N
9.	a	34.	K
10.	d	35.	A
11.	b	36.	B
12.	c	37.	D
13.	b	38.	I
14.	a	39.	G
15.	d	40.	C
16.	b	41.	AH
17.	b	42.	C-section, CS
18.	a	43.	D&C
19.	a	44.	EDC
20.	d	45.	FSH
21.	c	46.	Gyn
22.	a	47.	OB
23.	b	48.	LMP
24.	d	49.	PAP
25.	a	50.	PID

THE FEMALE REPRODUCTIVE SYSTEM
CHAPTER 15
POST TEST B

PART I WORD PARTS
DIRECTIONS: Using the answer sheet, write the letter of the definition that best matches the word part.

1. cata
2. multi
3. neo
4. nulli
5. primi
6. pseudo
7. cept
8. cervic
9. coit
10. colpo
11. episio
12. gyneco
13. hystero
14. mammo
15. meno
16. nata
17. oophor
18. partum
19. pause
20. pelvi
21. perineo
22. salpingo
23. venere
24. -cyesis
25. -genesis

A. breast
B. female
C. pelvis
D. receive
E. cessation
F. birth
G. vagina
H. first
I. formation
J. womb, uterus
K. vulva
L. none
M. pregnancy
N. new
O. many
P. down
Q. sexual intercourse
R. ovary
S. up
T. labor
U. a coming together
V. month
W. cervix
X. tube
Y. false
Z. perineum

PART II FILL-IN-THE-BLANK
DIRECTIONS: Using the answer sheet, write the correct abbreviation or meaning for each of the following.

26. AFP
27. CVS
28. dilation and curettage
29. diethylstilbestrol
30. EDC

31. GIFT
32. LMP
33. obstetrics
34. PID
35. PMS

PART III MULTIPLE CHOICE

DIRECTIONS: Select the best answer to each multiple choice question and write the appropriate letter on the answer sheet.

36. _____ is the act of giving birth.
    a. Pudendal   c. Quickening
    b. Puerperium   d. Parturition

37. A procedure that involves the insertion of a catheter into the cervix and into the outer portion of the membranes surrounding the fetus is called:
    a. amniotic fluid analysis
    b. chorionic villus sampling
    c. colposcopy
    d. culdoscopy

38. A positive result may indicate pregnancy.
    a. colposcopy   c. HCG
    b. culdoscopy   d. laparoscopy

39. X-ray of the uterus and fallopian tubes after the injection of a radiopaque substance.
    a. hysterosalpingography
    b. laparoscopy
    c. culdoscopy
    d. mammography

40. Used to examine the ovaries and fallopian tubes.
    a. colposcopy   c. laparoscopy
    b. culdoscopy   d. mammography

41. The process of obtaining pictures of the breast by use of x-rays.
    a. colposcopy   c. laparoscopy
    b. culdoscopy   d. mammography

42. The process in which an ovum is discharged from the cortex of the ovary is known as:
    a. mittelschmerz   c. quickening
    b. ovulation   d. menarche

43. The _____ is a musculomembranous tube extending from the vestibule to the uterus.
    a. ovary   c. fallopian tube
    b. eustachian tube   d. vagina

44. The following are identifiable areas of the uterus except:
    a. body   c. cortex
    b. isthmus   d. cervix

45. Finger-like processes that work to propel the discharged ovum into the tube are called:
    a. flagella   c. filum
    b. fimbriae   d. fillet

46. The process of bending forward of the uterus at its body and neck is called:
    a. anteflexion   c. anteversion
    b. retroflexion   d. retroversion

47. The external region between the vulva and the anus is:
    a. perineum   c. perineurium
    b. peritoneum   d. perinephrium

48. A woman who is bearing her first child is called:
    a. primipara   c. nullipara
    b. multipara   d. unipara

49. The male or female reproductive organs are called:
    a. genial   c. genal
    b. genetics   d. genitalia

50. Surgical excision of the uterus is:
    a. hysterotomy   c. hymenectomy
    b. hysterectomy   d. hysterorrhexis

THE FEMALE REPRODUCTIVE SYSTEM
CHAPTER 15
POST TEST B

ANSWER KEY:

1. P
2. O
3. N
4. L
5. H
6. Y
7. D
8. W
9. U
10. G
11. K
12. B
13. J
14. A
15. V
16. F
17. R
18. T
19. E
20. C
21. Z
22. X
23. Q
24. M
25. I

26. alpha-fetoprotein
27. chorionic villus sampling
28. D&C
29. DES
30. expected date of confinement
31. gamete intrafallopian transfer
32. last menstrual period
33. OB
34. pelvic inflammatory disease
35. premenstrual syndrome
36. d
37. b
38. c
39. a
40. c
41. d
42. b
43. d
44. c
45. b
46. a
47. a
48. a
49. d
50. b

THE MALE REPRODUCTIVE SYSTEM
CHAPTER 16
POST TEST A

PART I MULTIPLE CHOICE
DIRECTIONS: Select the best answer to each multiple choice question and write the appropriate letter on the answer sheet.

1. _____ is the loose skin folds that cover the penis.
   a. Glans penis   c. Smegma
   b. Prepuce   d. Rete testis

2. The site of the development of spermatozoa is:
   a. seminal vesicles   c. vas deferens
   b. epididymis   d. seminiferous tubules

3. Enlargement of the prostate that can occur in older men is:
   a. prostatic hypertrophy c. hypertrophy prostatic
   b. prostate trophy   d. megaloprostatic

4. The following are accessory glands of the male reproductive system except:
   a. seminal vesicles   c. bulbourethral
   b. testes   d. prostate

5. A lack of one or both testes is called:
   a. azoospermia   c. aorchism
   b. aspermatism   d. anorchism

6. Surgical process of removing the foreskin of the penis is:
   a. capacitation   c. circumcision
   b. castrate   d. circumflexion

7. Failure of the testis to descend into the scrotum is called:
   a. cryptorchism   c. cryptodidymus
   b. anorchism   d. cryptogenic

8. Congenital defect in which the urethra opens on the dorsum of the penis is called:
   a. epididymitis   c. epispadias
   b. hypospadias   d. hydrocele

9. Surgical fixation of a testicle is called:
   a. orchidectomy   c. orchidotomy
   b. orchidoplasty   d. orchidopexy

10. Surgical excision of a testicle is called:
    a. orchidectomy   c. orchidotomy
    b. orchidoplasty   d. orchidopexy

11. Inflammation of the prostate and bladder is called:
    a. prostatalgia   c. prostatitis
    b. prostatectomy   d. prostatocystitis

12. Enlargement and twisting of the veins of the spermatic cord
    is known as:
    a. vasectomy   c. vesiculitis
    b. varicocele   d. varicosity

13. An agent that kills sperm is a:
    a. spermatocyst   c. spermicide
    b. spermatoblast   d. spermaturia

14. The male sex cell is called:
    a. spermatozoon   c. spermatocyst
    b. spermatozoa   d. spermatolytic

15. Formation of spermatozoa is known as:
    a. spermaturia   c. spermatogenesis
    b. spermatocyst   d. spermatoblast

16. _____ is the surgical excision of the vas deferens.
    a. Vesiculitis   c. Vasotomy
    b. Varicocele   d. Vasectomy

17. Sexual intercourse between a man and a woman is called:
    a. coitus   c. castrate
    b. cloning   d. capacitation

18. The process of expulsion of seminal fluid from the male
    urethra is known as:
    a. eunuch   c. eugenics
    b. ejaculation   d. epispadias

19. A mature reproductive cell of the male or female is called:
    a. zygote   c. gamete
    b. mitosis   d. trisomy

20. A venereal disease caused by Treponema pallidum is:
    a. syphilis   c. herpes
    b. gonorrhea   d. AIDS

21. The prefix circum means:
    a. upon   c. around
    b. under   d. lack of

22. The word root crypt means:
    a. a rent   c. to pour
    b. hidden   d. seed

23. The suffix -cele means:
     a. to kill   c. hernia
     b. cell   d. condition of

24. The following terms are spelled correctly except for:
     a. hypospadias   c. spermaturia
     b. orchdotomy   d. prostatomegaly

25. Inflammation of the glans penis is known as:
     a. orchitis   c. vesiculitis
     b. prostatitis   d. balanitis

PART II MATCHING
DIRECTIONS: Using the answer sheet, write the letter of the definition that best matches the word.

26. hydrocele
27. orchidotomy
28. parenchyma
29. phimosis
30. trisomy
31. spermaturia
32. castrate
33. condyloma
34. cloning
35. condom
36. gonorrhea
37. gynecomastia
38. heterosexual
39. homosexual
40. infertility

A. Excessive development of the mammary glands in the male
B. A highly contagious venereal disease
C. To remove the testicles
D. Collection of serous fluid in a sac-like cavity
E. Discharge of semen with urine
F. Inability to produce a viable offspring
G. Incision into a testicle
H. Pertaining to the opposite sex
I. Pertaining to the same sex
J. Pertaining to being bisexual
K. Essential cells of a gland
L. Creating a genetic duplicate
M. Condition of a muzzle
N. A flexible, protective sheath
O. Having 3 chromosomes instead 2
P. A wart-like growth

PART III FILL-IN-THE-BLANK
DIRECTIONS: Using the answer sheet, write the correct abbreviation for each of the following.

41. _____ artificial insemination homologous
42. _____ benign prostatic hypertrophy
43. _____ herpes simplex virus-2
44. _____ suprapubic prostatectomy
45. _____ serologic test for syphilis
46. _____ Treponema pallidum agglutination
47. _____ transurethral resection
48. _____ urogenital
49. _____ venereal disease
50. _____ Wassermann reaction

ANSWER KEY:

1. b	26. D
2. d	27. G
3. a	28. K
4. b	29. M
5. d	30. O
6. c	31. E
7. a	32. C
8. c	33. P
9. d	34. L
10. a	35. N
11. d	36. B
12. b	37. A
13. c	38. H
14. a	39. I
15. c	40. F
16. d	41. AIH
17. a	42. BPH
18. b	43. HSV-2
19. c	44. SPP
20. a	45. STS
21. c	46. TPA
22. b	47. TUR
23. c	48. UG
24. b	49. VD
25. d	50. WR

THE MALE REPRODUCTIVE SYSTEM
CHAPTER 16
POST TEST B

PART I WORD PARTS
DIRECTIONS: Using the answer sheet, write the letter of the
definition that best matches the word part.

1. circum	A. life
2. epi	B. penis
3. oligo	C. to cut
4. par	D. hidden
5. balan	E. inflammation
6. cis	F. testicle
7. crypt	G. prostate
8. cyst	H. vessel
9. didym	I. twisted vein
10. enchyma	J. scanty
11. orchido	K. to pour
12. pen	L. animal
13. phim	M. process
14. prostato	N. glans
15. spadias	O. beside
16. spermato	P. around
17. varico	Q. to kill
18. vas	R. testis
19. vesicul	S. upon
20. zoo	T. hernia
21. zoon	U. vesicle
22. -cele	V. removal
23. -cide	W. a rent (opening)
24. -ion	X. a muzzle
25. -itis	Y. seed, sperm
	Z. bladder

PART II FILL-IN-THE-BLANK
DIRECTIONS: Using the answer sheet, write the correct
abbreviation or meaning for each of the following.

26. BPH
27. Gc
28. suprapubic prostatectomy
29. sexually transmitted
    diseases
30. TPA

31. TUR
32. urogenital
33. venereal disease
34. VDRL
35. WR

PART III MULTIPLE CHOICE

DIRECTIONS: Select the best answer to each multiple choice question and write the appropriate letter on the answer sheet.

36. The human papilloma virus (HPV) causes:
    a. chlamydia   c. gonorrhea
    b. genital warts   d. syphilis

37. Trichomoniasis is caused by a/an:
    a. protozoa   c. virus
    b. bacterium   d. fungus

38. Zovirax may be used to relieve symptoms of:
    a. gonorrhea   c. chlamydia
    b. syphilis   d. herpes genitalis

39. _____ is the loose skin folds that cover the penis.
    a. Glans penis   c. Smegma
    b. Prepuce   d. Rete testis

40. The site of the development of spermatozoa is:
    a. seminal vesicles   c. vas deferens
    b. epididymis   d. seminiferous tubules

41. Enlargement of the prostate that may occur in older men is:
    a. prostatic hypertrophy c. hypertrophy prostatic
    b. prostate trophy   d. megaloprostatic

42. Lack of one or both testes is called:
    a. azoospermia   c. aorchism
    b. aspermatism   d. anorchism

43. Surgical process of removing the foreskin of the penis is:
    a. capacitation   c. circumcision
    b. castrate   d. circumflex

44. Failure of the testis to descend into the scrotum is called:
    a. cryptorchism   c. cryptodidymus
    b. anorchism   d. cryptogenic

45. An agent that kills sperm is called:
    a. spermatocyst   c. spermicide
    b. spermatoblast   d. spermaturia

46. Increased level indicates prostate disease or possibly prostate cancer.
    a. fluorescent treponemal antibody
    b. prostate-specific antigen
    c. semen
    d. testosterone

47. Used to determine infertility in the male.
    a. paternity
    b. prostate-specific antigen
    c. semen
    d. testosterone toxicology

48. Increased level may indicate benign prostatic hypertrophy.
    a. fluorescent treponemal antibody
    b. prostate-specific antigen
    c. testosterone toxicology
    d. venereal disease research

49. A test performed on blood serum to detect syphilis.
    a. paternity   c. FTA-ABS
    b. semen   d. HSV-2

50. Test to determine whether a certain person could be the
    father of a specific child.
    a. paternity   c. FTA-ABS
    b. semen   d. HSV-2

THE MALE REPRODUCTIVE SYSTEM
CHAPTER 16
POST TEST B

ANSWER KEY:

1. P
2. S
3. J
4. O
5. N
6. C
7. D
8. Z
9. R
10. K
11. F
12. B
13. X
14. G
15. W
16. Y
17. I
18. H
19. U
20. L
21. A
22. T
23. Q
24. M
25. E

26. benign prostatic hypertrophy
27. gonorrhea
28. SPP
29. STDs
30. Treponema pallidum agglutination
31. transurethral resection
32. UG
33. VD
34. venereal disease research laboratory
35. Wassermann reaction
36. b
37. a
38. d
39. b
40. d
41. a
42. d
43. c
44. a
45. c
46. b
47. c
48. c
49. c
50. a

ONCOLOGY
CHAPTER 17
POST TEST A

PART I MULTIPLE CHOICE
DIRECTIONS: Select the best answer to each multiple choice
question and write the appropriate letter on the answer sheet.

1. The process whereby normal cells have a distinct appearance
    and specialized function is:
    a. mitosis   c. dedifferentiation
    b. anaplasia   d. differentiation

2. The following are ways that malignant cells spread to body
    parts except for:
    a. active migration   c. metastasis
    b. direct extension   d. effusion

3. A _____ is any agent or substance that incites cancer.
    a. carcinogen   c. carcinoid
    b. carcinoma   d. carcinomatosis

4. Cancer causing genes are known as:
    a. oncogenics   c. onocogenes
    b. oncolytics   d. oncogenes

5. A cancerous tumor of a gland is:
    a. carcinoadenoma   c. astrocytoma
    b. adenocarcinoma   d. glioma

6. A cancerous tumor originating from blood vessels is:
    a. hemangiosarcoma   c. fibrosarcoma
    b. angiohemosarcoma   d. choriocarcinoma

7. Excessive formation and growth of normal cells is:
    a. hypercalcemia   c. hyperplasia
    b. hypercyesis   d. hyperhidrosis

8. A disease of the blood characterized by overproduction of
    leukocytes is called:
    a. leukoplakia   c. liposarcoma
    b. leukemia   d. lymphoma

9. A _____ is a cancerous black mole or tumor.
    a. melanoma   c. neoplasm
    b. myeloma   d. melanoblast

10. A cancerous tumor arising from connective tissue is called:
    a. carcinoma   c. sarcoma
    b. mixed cancer   d. lymphoma

11. The medical term _____ means the inability to open the mouth fully.
    a. stomatitis   c. violaceous
    b. scirrhus   d. trismus

12. The process of lessening the severity of symptoms is:
    a. exacerbation   c. proliferation
    b. remission   d. invasive

13. A cancerous tumor of the kidney occurring mainly in children is called:
    a. glioblastoma   c. Wilm's tumor
    b. hypernephroma   d. teratoma

14. The prefix ana means:
    a. lack of   c. before
    b. up   d. after

15. The combining form immuno means:
    a. fiber   c. safe
    b. gland   d. net

16. The combining form leio means:
    a. smooth   c. soft
    b. hard   d. white

17. The suffix -blast means:
    a. formation   c. produce
    b. immature cell   d. pertaining to

18. The American Cancer Society list _____ warning signals for cancer.
    a. six   c. seven
    b. five   d. eight

19. The following are characteristics of malignant tumors except:
    a. grow rapidly
    b. encapsulated
    c. spread via the blood stream
    d. cells undergo permanent change

20. Surgical removal of a small piece of tissue for microscopic examination is known as:
    a. pap smear   c. biopsy
    b. Hemoccult   d. endoscopy

21. The first virus known to cause cancer is humans is:
    a. human B-cell leukemia-lymphoma virus
    b. human T-cell leukemia-lymphoma virus
    c. T-lymphocytoma virus
    d. herpes zoster

22. The process whereby the genetic structure is changed is:
    a. mutation   c. malignant
    b. mutagen   d. metastasis

23. A cancerous tumor derived from cartilage cells is:
    a. sarcochondroma   c. carcinoma
    b. choriocarcinoma   d. chondrosarcoma

24. Treatment of disease by active, passive or adoptive immunity is called:
    a. chemotherapy   c. immunotherapy
    b. radiotherapy   d. imunotherapy

25. A cancerous tumor of fat cells is called:
    a. sarcolipoma   c. adiposoma
    b. liposarcoma   d. lipoadipoma

PART II MATCHING
DIRECTIONS: Using the answer sheet, write the letter of the definition that best matches the word(s).

26. Hodgkin's disease
27. exacerbation
28. differentiation
29. in situ
30. interleukin-2
31. photodynamic therapy
32. recombinant interferon
33. tumor necrosis factor
34. Kaposi's sarcoma
35. malignant
36. xerostomia
37. lesion
38. encapsulated
39. palliative
40. proliferation

A. Enclosed within a sheath
B. The spreading process of cancer from one area of the body to another
C. Rapid reproduction
D. Lymphokine produced by macrophages
E. Dryness of mouth
F. Genetically engineered immune-boosting drug
G. Relieve or alleviate symptoms
H. The process whereby normal cells have a distinct appearance and specialized function
I. A form of lymphoma that occurs in young adults
J. A wound
K. Use of a red laser to kill cancerous cells
L. To stay within a site
M. Malignant neoplasm that causes violaceous vascular lesions
N. Process of increasing the severity of symptoms
O. Genetically engineered immune system activator
P. Agent that causes a change in the genetic structure of an organism

PART III FILL-IN-THE-BLANK
DIRECTIONS: Using the answer sheet, write the correct abbreviation or meaning for each of the following.

41. _____ adenocarcinoma
42. _____ biopsy
43. _____ CA
44. _____ chem
45. _____ deoxyribonucleic acid
46. _____ IL-2
47. _____ lymphokine-activated killer
48. _____ Mets
49. _____ TNF
50. _____ TNM

ONCOLOGY
CHAPTER 17
POST TEST A

ANSWER KEY:

1.	d	26.	I
2.	d	27.	N
3.	a	28.	H
4.	d	29.	L
5.	b	30.	F
6.	a	31.	K
7.	c	32.	O
8.	b	33.	D
9.	a	34.	M
10.	c	35.	B
11.	d	36.	E
12.	b	37.	J
13.	c	38.	A
14.	b	39.	G
15.	c	40.	C
16.	a	41.	Adeno-Ca
17.	b	42.	Bx
18.	c	43.	cancer
19.	b	44.	chemotherapy
20.	c	45.	DNA
21.	b	46.	interleukin-2
22.	a	47.	LAK
23.	d	48.	metastases
24.	c	49.	tumor necrosis factor
25.	b	50.	tumor, node, metastasis

ONCOLOGY
CHAPTER 17
POST TEST B

PART I WORD PARTS

DIRECTIONS: Using the answer sheet, write the letter of the definition that best matches the word part.

1. ana
2. astro
3. neo
4. carcino
5. chorio
6. dendro
7. fibro
8. gli
9. immuno
10. leuko
11. leio
12. medullo
13. melan
14. onco
15. sarco
16. terat
17. tox
18. trism
19. xero
20. -genes
21. -ous
22. -plakia
23. -plasia
24. -plasm
25. -therapy

A. tree
B. tumor
C. safe
D. poison
E. up
F. produce
G. formation
H. plate
I. chorion
J. marrow
K. a thing formed
L. white
M. star-shaped
N. flesh
O. fiber
P. glue
Q. pertaining to
R. treatment
S. new
T. cancer
U. black
V. tumor
W. smooth
X. monster
Y. dry
Z. grating

PART II FILL-IN-THE-BLANK

DIRECTIONS: Using the answer sheet, write the correct abbreviation or meaning for each of the following.

26. BX
27. cancer
28. chem
29. DNA
30. Hodgkin's disease
31. interleukin-2
32. Mets
33. RNA
34. tumor necrosis factor
35. TNM

PART III MULTIPLE CHOICE
DIRECTIONS: Select the best answer to each multiple choice
question and write the appropriate letter on the answer sheet.

36. The process whereby normal cells have a distinct appearance
    and specialized function is:
    a. mitosis   c. dedifferentiation
    b. anaplasia   d. differentiation

37. The following are ways that malignant cells spread to body
    parts except for:
    a. active migration   c. metastasis
    b. direct extension   d. effusion

38. A _____ is any agent or substance that incites cancer.
    a. carcinogen   c. carcinoid
    b. carcinoma   d. carcinolysis

39. Cancer causing genes are known as:
    a. oncogenics   c. onocogenes
    b. oncolytics   d. oncogenes

40. A cancerous tumor of a gland is called:
    a. carcinoadenoma   c. astrocytoma
    b. adenocarcinoma   d. glioma

41. A cancerous tumor originating from blood vessels is:
    a. hemangiosarcoma   c. fibrosarcoma
    b. angiohemosarcoma   d. choriocarcinoma

42. Excessive formation and growth of normal cells is:
    a. hypercalcemia   c. hyperplasia
    b. hypercyesis   d. hyperhidrosis

43. A disease of the blood characterized by overproduction of
    leukocytes is:
    a. leukoplakia   c. liposarcoma
    b. leukemia   d. lymphoma

44. A _____ is a cancerous black mole or tumor.
    a. melanoma   c. neoplasm
    b. myeloma   d. melanoblast

45. A cancerous tumor arising from connective tissue is:
    a. carcinoma   c. sarcoma
    b. mixed cancer   d. lymphoma

46. The medical term for inability to open the mouth fully is:
    a. stomatitis   c. violaceous
    b. scirrhus   d. trismus

47. The process of lessening the severity of symptoms is:
   a. exacerbation   c. proliferation
   b. remission   d. invasive

48. A cancerous tumor of the kidney occurring mainly in children is called:
   a. glioblastoma   c. Wilm's tumor
   b. hypernephroma   d. teratoma

49. The following are characteristics of malignant tumors except for:
   a. grow rapidly
   b. encapsulated
   c. spread via the blood stream
   d. cells undergo permanent change

50. Surgical removal of a small piece of tissue for microscopic examination is known as:
   a. pap smear   c. biopsy
   b. Hemoccult   d. endoscopy

ONCOLOGY
CHAPTER 17
POST TEST B

ANSWER KEY:

1.	E	26.	biopsy
2.	M	27.	CA
3.	S	28.	chemotherapy
4.	T	29.	deoxyribonucleic acid
5.	I	30.	HD
6.	A	31.	IL-2
7.	O	32.	metastases
8.	P	33.	ribonucleic acid
9.	C	34.	TNF
10.	L	35.	tumor, node, metastasis
11.	W	36.	d
12.	J	37.	d
13.	U	38.	a
14.	B	39.	d
15.	N	40.	b
16.	X	41.	a
17.	D	42.	c
18.	Z	43.	b
19.	Y	44.	a
20.	F	45.	c
21.	Q	46.	d
22.	H	47.	b
23.	G	48.	c
24.	K	49.	b
25.	R	50.	c

RADIOLOGY AND NUCLEAR MEDICINE
CHAPTER 18
POST TEST A

PART I MULTIPLE CHOICE
DIRECTIONS: Select the best answer to each multiple choice
question and write the appropriate letter on the answer sheet.

1. All of the following are characteristics of x-rays except:
   a. invisible form of radiant energy
   b. long wave lengths
   c. cause ionization
   d. excite fluorescence

2. All of the following are dangers of x-rays except:
   a. depresses the heart rate
   b. depresses the hematopoietic system
   c. damage to the gonads
   d. causes leukemia

3. All of the following are safety precautions designed to
   prevent unnecessary exposure to x-rays except:
   a. wearing a film badge
   b. using protective clothing
   c. standing behind an unleaded screen
   d. using a gonad shield

4. The process of making an x-ray record of blood vessels is:
   a. angiogram   c. aortogram
   b. angiocardiogram   d. angiography

5. Radiation therapy where the radioactive substance is inserted
   into a body cavity or organ is known as:
   a. bradytherapy   c. teletherapy
   b. brachytherapy   d. radiotherapy

6. The process of using ultrasound as a diagnostic tool is:
   a. fluoroscopy   c. echography
   b. holography   d. radiography

7. The process of obtaining pictures of the breast through the
   use of x-rays is:
   a. mammography   c. mastography
   b. mammogram   d. mastogram

8. One who is skilled in making x-rays is called a:
   a. radiograph   c. radiology
   b. radiographer   d. radiogenic

9. One who specializes in radiology is called a:
   a. radiologist   c. dosimetrist
   b. oncologist   d. physicist

151

10. The property of permitting the passage of radiant energy is:
    a. radiopaque   c. radiolucent
    b. radioactive   d. radiogenic

11. A record produced by ultrasonography is called:
    a. thermogram   c. angiogram
    b. mammogram   d. sonogram

12. The process of cutting across and producing images of single tissue planes is:
    a. thermography   c. sonography
    b. tomography   d. mammography

13. The medical term for pertaining to hair loss is:
    a. anorexia   c. alopecia
    b. artifact   d. anemia

14. A light-proof case or holder for x-ray film is called:
    a. cassette   c. collimator
    b. cathode   d. cone

15. A unit of radioactivity is known as:
    a. atom   c. curie
    b. ion   d. rad

16. A charge or unit of negative electricity that revolves around the nucleus of an atom is:
    a. proton   c. neutron
    b. electron   d. betatron

17. In radiation therapy, a _____ refers to the skin area of entry for the radiation.
    a. port   c. beam
    b. dose   d. ampere

18. All of the following are diagnostic tools that may be used in radiology except for:
    a. computed tomography   c. thermography
    b. external radiation   d. nuclear magnetic resonance

19. The prefix brachy means:
    a. short   c. long
    b. slow   d. fast

20. The combining form cinemato means:
    a. distant   c. motion
    b. sound   d. light

21. The suffix -graphy means:
    a. record   c. instrument
    b. recording   d. to view

22. An x-ray record of the gallbladder is called:
    a. cholecystography   c. cholangiogram
    b. cholecystectomy   d. cholecystogram

23. All of the following are spelled correctly except for:
    a. sialography   c. venography
    b. myelogram   d. pneumencephalgram

24. Treatment by introducing ions into the body is called:
    a. ionometer   c. ionotherapy
    b. ionoradiometer   d. iontherapy

25. An x-ray record of the kidney and renal pelvis is called:
    a. intravenous pyelogram
    b. intervenous pyelogram
    c. intravenous pyelography
    d. venous pyelogram

PART II MATCHING
DIRECTIONS: Using the answer sheet, write the letter of the
definition that best matches the word.

26. anode
27. beam
28. kilovolt
29. contrast medium
30. energy
31. in vitro
32. lead
33. rad
34. tagging
35. watt
36. venography
37. radioactive
38. radionecrosis
39. thermography
40. aplastic anemia

A. A ray of light
B. One thousand volts
C. Emitting radiant energy
D. Death of tissue caused by
    exposure to radiant energy
E. Positive pole of an electrical
    current
F. An anemia with aplasia or
    destruction of bone marrow
G. Process of recording heat
    patterns of the body's surface
H. Radiopaque substance
I. The capacity to do work
J. Within a glass
K. A metallic, chemical element
L. Amount of radiation absorbed
M. Unit of electrical power
N. Tracing a radioactive isotope
O. Process of making an x-ray
    image of veins
P. Process of using ultrasound

PART III FILL-IN-THE-BLANK
DIRECTIONS: Using the answer sheet, write the correct abbreviation for each of the following.

41. _____ anteroposterior
42. _____ barium enema
43. _____ computed tomography
44. _____ kilowatt
45. _____ milliampere
46. _____ millicurie
47. _____ radiation absorbed dose
48. _____ nuclear magnetic resonance
49. _____ pneumoencephalogram
50. _____ positron emission tomography

RADIOLOGY AND NUCLEAR MEDICINE
CHAPTER 18
POST TEST A

ANSWER KEY:

1.	b		26.	E
2.	a		27.	A
3.	c		28.	B
4.	d		29.	H
5.	b		30.	I
6.	c		31.	J
7.	a		32.	K
8.	b		33.	L
9.	a		34.	N
10.	c		35.	M
11.	d		36.	O
12.	b		37.	C
13.	c		38.	D
14.	a		39.	G
15.	c		40.	F
16.	b		41.	AP
17.	a		42.	BaE
18.	b		43.	CT
19.	a		44.	KW
20.	c		45.	Ma
21.	b		46.	MC
22.	d		47.	rad
23.	d		48.	NMR
24.	c		49.	PEG
25.	a		50.	PET

RADIOLOGY AND NUCLEAR MEDICINE
CHAPTER 18
POST TEST B

PART I WORD PARTS
DIRECTIONS: Using the answer sheet, write the letter of the definition that best matches the word part.

1.	brachy	A.	death
2.	milli	B.	cavity
3.	ultra	C.	to cut
4.	cavit	D.	pertaining to
5.	cinemato	E.	dark
6.	dosi	F.	one-thousandth
7.	electro	G.	heat
8.	fluoro	H.	short
9.	holo	I.	sound
10.	iono	J.	to swing
11.	kilo	K.	nature of
12.	necr	L.	beyond
13.	oscillo	M.	salivary
14.	paque	N.	motion
15.	photo	O.	a giving
16.	radio	P.	process
17.	roent	Q.	electricity
18.	sialo	R.	recording
19.	sono	S.	fluorescence
20.	thermo	T.	ion
21.	tomo	U.	ray
22.	-ary	V.	whole
23.	-graphy	W.	one-thousand
24.	-ion	X.	light
25.	-ive	Y.	roentgen
		Z.	vein

PART II FILL-IN-THE-BLANK
DIRECTIONS: Using the answer sheet, write the correct abbreviation or meaning for each of the following.

26.	AP	31.	pneumoencephalogram
27.	BaE	32.	radiation absorbed dose
28.	computed tomography	33.	PET
29.	IRT	34.	NMR
30.	LL	35.	posteroanterior

PART III MULTIPLE CHOICE
DIRECTIONS: Select the best answer to each multiple choice question and write the appropriate letter on the answer sheet.

36. The property of permitting the passage of radiant energy is:
    a. radiopaque   c. radiolucent
    b. radioactive   d. radiogenic

37. A record produced by ultrasonography is called:
    a. thermogram   c. angiogram
    b. mammogram   d. sonogram

38. The process of cutting across and producing images of single tissue planes is:
    a. thermography   c. sonography
    b. tomography   d. mammography

39. The medical term for pertaining to hair loss is:
    a. anorexia   c. alopecia
    b. artifact   d. anemia

40. A light-proof case or holder for x-ray film is called:
    a. cassette   c. collimator
    b. cathode   d. cone

41. A unit of radioactivity is known as:
    a. atom   c. curie
    b. ion   d. rad

42. A charge or unit of negative electricity that revolves around the nucleus of an atom is:
    a. proton   c. neutron
    b. electron   d. betatron

43. In radiation therapy, a _____ refers to the skin area of entry for the radiation.
    a. port   c. beam
    b. dose   d. ampere

44. All of the following are diagnostic tools that may be used in radiology except for:
    a. computed tomography   c. thermography
    b. external radiation   d. nuclear magnetic resonance

45. The prefix brachy means:
    a. short   c. long
    b. slow   d. fast

46. The combining form cinemato means:
    a. distant   c. motion
    b. sound   d. light

47. The suffix -graphy means:
    a. record   c. instrument
    b. recording   d. to view

48. An x-ray record of the gallbladder is called:
    a. cholecystography   c. cholangiogram
    b. cholecystectomy   d. cholecystogram

49. All of the following are spelled correctly except for:
    a. sialography   c. venography
    b. myelogram   d. pneumencephalgram

50. Treatment by introducing ions into the body is called:
    a. ionometer   c. ionotherapy
    b. ionoradiometer   d. iontherapy

RADIOLOGY AND NUCLEAR MEDICINE
CHAPTER 18
POST TEST B

ANSWER KEY:

1.	H	26.	anteroposterior
2.	F	27.	barium enema
3.	L	28.	CT
4.	B	29.	internal radiation therapy
5.	N	30.	left lateral
6.	O	31.	PEG
7.	Q	32.	rad
8.	S	33.	positron emission tomography
9.	V	34.	nuclear magnetic resonance
10.	T	35.	PA
11.	W	36.	c
12.	A	37.	d
13.	J	38.	b
14.	E	39.	c
15.	X	40.	a
16.	U	41.	c
17.	Y	42.	b
18.	M	43.	a
19.	I	44.	b
20.	G	45.	a
21.	C	46.	c
22.	D	47.	b
23.	R	48.	d
24.	P	49.	d
25.	K	50.	c

PART I MULTIPLE CHOICE
DIRECTIONS: Select the best answer to each multiple choice question and write the appropriate letter on the answer sheet.

1. A syllable placed at the beginning of a word is called a/an:
   a. suffix
   b. root
   c. prefix
   d. combining form

2. The foundation of a word is the:
   a. combining vowel
   b. combining form
   c. word root
   d. prefix

3. The _____ plane divides the body into superior and inferior portions:
   a. coronal
   b. midsagittal
   c. frontal
   d. transverse

4. The prefix ambi means:
   a. double
   b. two
   c. both
   d. one

5. Excessive flow of oil from the sebaceous glands is called:
   a. sebolite
   b. hidrosis
   c. hidrorrhea
   d. seborrhea

6. A physician may refer to a scar left after the healing of a wound as a:
   a. cicatrix
   b. comedo
   c. corn
   d. crust

7. A condition that results in reduction of bone mass is called:
   a. osteoporosis
   b. osteopenia
   c. osteonecrosis
   d. osteofibroma

8. A lateral curvature of the spine is known as:
   a. lordosis
   b. kyphosis
   c. scoliosis
   d. scoliotone

9. The prefix syn means:
   a. separate
   b. joined
   c. apart
   d. together

10. The combining form acro means:
    a. crooked
    b. extremity
    c. joint
    d. bone

11. The word root chondr means:
    a. cancer
    b. clavicle
    c. glue
    d. cartilage

12. A condition in which there is an abnormal darkening of muscle tissue is:
    a. myoparesis   c. myorrhaphy
    b. myomelanosis   d. myorrhexis

13. The combining form quadri means:
    a. four   c. three
    b. two   d. six

14. The study of the stomach and the intestine is:
    a. gastrology   c. gastroenterology
    b. enterology   d. enterogastrology

15. _____ is inflammation of the liver.
    a. Hepatoma   c. Nephroma
    b. Nephritis   d. Hepatitis

16. A condition in which the colon is extremely enlarged is:
    a. diverticulitis   c. enteritis
    b. megacolon   d. microcolon

17. The _____ _____ is located in the antecubital space of the elbow.
    a. radial pulse   c. carotid pulse
    b. brachial pulse   d. femoral pulse

18. The most common site for taking a pulse is the _____ artery.
    a. carotid   c. brachial
    b. femoral   d. radial

19. The medical term for a tumor of the thymus is:
    a. thymitis   c. thymoma
    b. thymocyte   d. thrombosis

20. A blood enzyme which causes clotting by forming fibrin is:
    a. thromboplastin   c. heparin
    b. fibrinogen   d. thrombin

21. The medical term for whooping cough is:
    a. pleurisy   c. polyp
    b. pertussis   d. rale

22. _____ _____ is the amount of air in a single inspiration or expiration.
    a. Residual volume   c. Total capacity
    b. Vital capacity   d. Tidal volume

23. All of the following terms refer to the process of emptying the bladder except:
    a. micturition   c. void
    b. urochrome   d. urination

24. The normal color of urine is:
    a. red   c. yellow to amber
    b. orange   d. greenish-yellow

25. Under chemical examination, the presence of _____ in the urine is an important sign of renal disease, acute glomerulonephritis and pyelonephritis.
    a. glucose   c. bilirubin
    b. protein   d. nitrites

PART II MATCHING
DIRECTIONS: Using the answer sheet, write the letter of the definition that best matches the word.

26. adenoma
27. adrenal
28. diabetes
29. gigantism
30. hirsutism
31. hyperkalemia
32. hypogonadism
33. oxytocin
34. parathyroid
35. thyroid
36. virilism
37. vasopressin
38. epinephrine
39. dwarfism
40. testosterone

A. Also called ADH
B. A condition of being abnormally small
C. Stimulates uterine contraction during childbirth
D. A condition of being abnormally large
E. Excessive amounts of potassium in the blood
F. A tumor of a gland
G. Also called adrenaline
H. Toward the kidney
I. Male sex hormone
J. Masculinity developed in a female
K. Hairy condition
L. Literally means "to go through"
M. Deficient internal secretion of the gonads
N. Located beside the thyroid gland
O. Resembling a shield
P. Masculinity developed in a male

PART III FILL-IN-THE-BLANK
DIRECTIONS: Using the answer sheet, write the correct abbreviation for each of the following.

41. _____ amyotrophic lateral sclerosis
42. _____ chronic brain syndrome
43. _____ cerebral palsy
44. _____ cerebrovascular accident
45. _____ electroencephalogram
46. _____ herniated disk syndrome
47. _____ intracranial pressure
48. _____ mental retardation
49. _____ nerve conduction velocity
50. _____ pneumoencephalography

MEDICAL TERMINOLOGY
POST TEST A - FINAL

ANSWER KEY:

1.	c	26.	F
2.	c	27.	H
3.	d	28.	L
4.	c	29.	D
5.	d	30.	K
6.	a	31.	E
7.	a	32.	M
8.	c	33.	C
9.	d	34.	N
10.	b	35.	O
11.	d	36.	J
12.	b	37.	A
13.	a	38.	G
14.	c	39.	B
15.	d	40.	I
16.	b	41.	ALS
17.	b	42.	CBS
18.	d	43.	CP
19.	c	44.	CVA
20.	d	45.	EEG
21.	b	46.	HDS
22.	d	47.	ICP
23.	b	48.	MR
24.	c	49.	NCV
25.	b	50.	PEG

MEDICAL TERMINOLOGY
POST TEST B - FINAL

PART I WORD PARTS
DIRECTIONS: Using the answer sheet, write the letter of the definition that best matches the word part.

1. ambi
2. ana
3. bi
4. chromo
5. de
6. ecto
7. endo
8. homeo
9. meso
10. proto
11. uni
12. adip
13. andr
14. cyt
15. histo
16. hydr
17. karyo
18. patho
19. physio
20. -ate
21. -logy
22. -oid
23. -some
24. -stasis
25. -tomy

A. outside
B. first
C. study of
D. body
E. both
F. fat
G. man
H. color
I. resemble
J. control
K. tissue
L. up
M. water
N. within
O. disease
P. two
Q. nature
R. middle
S. use, action
T. excision
U. down
V. one
W. incision
X. similar
Y. cell
Z. cell's nucleus

PART II FILL-IN-THE-BLANK
DIRECTIONS: Using the answer sheet, write the correct abbreviation or meaning for each of the following.

26. abnormal
27. ac
28. Bx
29. Dx
30. D/C

31. gram
32. Gyn
33. liter
34. mL
35. DRGs

PART III MULTIPLE CHOICE
DIRECTIONS: Select the best answer to each multiple choice question and write the appropriate letter on the answer sheet.

36. Amyotrophic lateral sclerosis is also known as:
    a. apoplexy   c. autism
    b. Lou Gehrig's disease d. Alzheimer's disease

37. _____ are chemical substances that act as natural analgesics.
    a. Acetylcholines   c. Endorphins
    b. Biogenic amines   d. Receptors

38. The medical term for fainting is:
    a. sciatica   c. narcolepsy
    b. syncope   d. palsy

39. The _____ nervous system consists of the brain and spinal cord.
    a. peripheral   c. autonomic
    b. central   d. sympathetic

40. All of the following membranes enclose the brain except:
    a. dura mater   c. pia mater
    b. arachnoid   d. oblongata

41. Which lobe is the brain's major motor area?
    a. parietal   c. temporal
    b. frontal   d. occipital

42. An instrument used to measure hearing is called:
    a. otoscope   c. audiometer
    b. audiphone   d. myringoscope

43. The clear fluid contained within the labyrinth is called:
    a. perilymph   c. plasma
    b. cerumen   d. endolymph

44. The process of sharpening the focus of light on the retina is known as:
    a. vision   c. accommodation
    b. contraction   d. dilation

45. The anterior transparent portion of the eyeball is the:
    a. sclera   c. retina
    b. cornea   d. iris

46. The process of bending forward of the uterus at its body and neck is called:
    a. anteflexion   c. anteversion
    b. retroflexion d. retroversion

47. The external region between the vulva and the anus is:
    a. perineum   c. perineurium
    b. peritoneum   d. perinephrium

48. Increased level may indicate benign prostatic hypertrophy.
    a. fluorescent treponemal antibody
    b. prostate-specific antigen
    c. testosterone toxicology
    d. venereal disease research

49. A test performed on blood serum to detect syphilis.
    a. paternity   c. FTA-ABS
    b. semen   d. HSV-2

50. Test to determine whether a certain person could be the
    father of a specific child.
    a. paternity   c. FTA-ABS
    b. semen   d. HSV-2

MEDICAL TERMINOLOGY
POST TEST B - FINAL

ANSWER KEY:

1. E
2. L
3. P
4. H
5. U
6. A
7. N
8. X
9. R
10. B
11. V
12. F
13. G
14. Y
15. K
16. M
17. Z
18. O
19. Q
20. S
21. C
22. I
23. D
24. J
25. W

26. AB
27. acute
28. biopsy
29. diagnosis
30. discontinue
31. g, Gm
32. gynecology
33. L
34. milliliter
35. diagnosis related groups
36. b
37. c
38. b
39. b
40. d
41. b
42. c
43. d
44. c
45. b
46. a
47. a
48. c
49. c
50. a